Pendulum
Healing
Handbook

Walter Lübeck

Pendulum
Healing
Handbook

Complete Guidebook on How to Use the Pendulum
to Choose Appropriate Remedies
for Healing Body, Mind, and Spirit

Translated by Christine M. Grimm

LOTUS PRESS
SHANGRI-LA

The information and exercises preented in this book have been carefully researched and passed on to the best of the author's knowledge and conscience. Despite this fact, the author and publisher do not assume any type of liability for damages of any type resulting directly or indirectly from the application or utilization of information given in this book. Naturally you should see a medical professionell if there is—or there should be—a serious illness!

4th printing 2012
3rd printing 2006
2nd printing 1999
1st English edition 1998
© Lotus Press
P.O. Box 325
Twin Lakes, WI 53181 USA
www.lotuspress.com
lotuspress@lotuspress.com
The Shangri-La Series is published in cooperation
with Windpferd Verlagsgesellschaft mbH, Federal Republic of Germany
© 1992 reserved by Windpferd Verlagsgesellschaft mbH, Oberstdorf
All rights reserved
Translated by Christine M. Grimm
Layout: *panta rhei!* – MediaServce Uwe Hiltmann

ISBN-13: 978-0-9149-5554-2   ISBN-10: 0-9149-5554-3
Library of Congress Number 97-76439

Printed in the USA

TABLE OF CONTENTS

Introduction

For many years now, the pendulum has been a good friend and helper to me on my journeys of discovery into the spiritual world with its many different types of energies. Like many other people, and perhaps like yourself as well as you read these lines, I have often asked myself the question of how and why it most likely works so often and why it sometimes doesn't, why some people are successful at it and why the pendulum behaves as if it were frozen for others. A great many books about how to use the pendulum have therefore found their way from the bookstore to my bedside table. I've also had long hours of interesting conversations with pendulum pros and radiesthetists, people involved in the theory and practice of using the pendulum, dowsing rods, and related areas, which have enriched my knowledge in this field—however, without actually being able to give me conclusive rules for the "how" and "why" of using the pendulum.

Later, after I had been initiated into Second Degree Reiki and experimented in the following period of time a great deal with the fantastic possibilities of this method of advanced energy work, things came together quickly and I understood what allows the pendulum to function, what its possibilities and limitations are, and how people for whom the pendulum doesn't work at first can rediscover this ability. Since, as far as I know, there is currently no book that explains these correlations in a way that is conclusive and easily understandable for beginners, I decided to write one. In my opinion, the work with the pendulum and the reasons why and how it functions are too important for them to just be known to the small circle of "initiates."

When you go on a journey of discovery in the land of energies with this book, on the basis of my experience I recommend that you do the very basic exercises time and again in order to expand and test your own abilities. Even if you are an "old hand" when it comes to using the pendulum, you still shouldn't skip over the introductory chapter. Although it introduces the ABCs, it still includes many important things that can be a big help to you and that you possibly won't find out about anywhere else.

I have included many pendulum tables that have been tested in everyday practice, along with explanations and references to more detailed literature so that you won't have to "invent the wheel" once again yourself. So you can just get started, if you want. If you would like to make your own pendulum tables, you will find instructions on the best way to make them and how to get the most benefit from them in a special chapter.

The more you work with the pendulum, the more important the theoretical background will be. Without it, you can hardly do extensive and truly profound pendulum work. I personally have an increasingly hard time learning theoretical things by heart. If you have the same problem, then simply look at the theory chapter whenever you aren't sure of how to proceed. Perhaps you will find the stories there so interesting that you just keep on reading ...

So, now I don't want to keep you from using the pendulum any longer! Take it out and get to work!

I wish you much enjoyment with it!

Walter Fülöp

CHAPTER 1

FUNDAMENTAL CONCEPTS OF USING THE PENDULUM

Let's start with the ABCs and first clarify some of the basic circumstances. For example:

WHAT DOES USING THE PENDULUM MEAN AND HOW DOES IT WORK?

In the area of radiesthesia, the expression of subtle-energetic perceptions by means of a pendulum held with the hand, meaning a flexible connection (string, chain, or something similar) on which a weighted object (mason's plumb bob, tip of a nail, crystal, etc.) is attached is called using the pendulum. In simple terms: when you hold one end of a necklace with a quartz-crystal pendant and the quartz crystal hangs downwards, you have a pendulum.

Working with the pendulum functions because your body has extremely keen senses that constantly take in a great deal of information on the subtle level. This is passed on to your subconscious mind and can be transmitted to your conscious mind by way of fine, unconscious reactions by the musculature as the pendulum's oscillations. What's actually so wonderful about the whole thing is then not so much the, admittedly impressive, oscillations of the pendulum in your hand but your body, which has the possibility of perceiving the many subtle vibrations and thereby causing such differentiated reactions in the musculature. Perhaps the question why a pendulum is necessary at all and whether the matter couldn't also function on its own may now occur to you. Your idea is right, things really do work without it! However, this requires certain processes of increasing consciousness, training, and practice!

But let's keep things as simple as possible in this book and learn to work with the pendulum, this wonderful instrument that can be a good companion for you on your journey of discovery into the world of subtle energies and an important adviser in the problems of everyday life.

WHAT SHOULD YOU USE AS A PENDULUM?

Today you can get pendulums in hundreds of forms from many esoteric bookshops and mail-order companies. Don't let yourself be confused by the silver cups, gold plating, particularly crystals and the like that are often recommended as especially suitable. Not everything that glitters is gold and also not everything that is expensive and unusual is useful. During my long "career in using the pendulum," I have worked with both purchased brass, silver, gold, and crystal pendulums in a great variety of forms, as well as with homemade pendulums with pendulum bodies made of sawed-off nail tips, different types of wood pieces, screw nuts, screws, pebbles, and the like. All of them functioned equally well, as long as the pendulum body was halfway rotationally symmetrical and I treated it in a sensible way. In some situations, I absolutely needed information from a pendulum but unfortunately didn't have one along with me. In these cases, "emergency pendulums" like bath brushes with a hanging loop, key chains, nails, or fat paperclips often helped me. This is just an example to make it easier for you to free yourself from preconceptions regarding the suitability of certain objects as pendulums, in as far as you have these.

There are basically just five criteria for a good pendulum:

a) A flexible connector (silk or cotton thread, but a thin metal necklace is better because it's sturdier) of about 20 centimeters in length.[1]

b) A rotationally symmetrical pendulum body must be attached to the flexible connector. This should be as pointed at the bottom as possible in order for you to work with it precisely, above all with the pendulum tables. For determining a pure oscillation pattern (for example, yes/no; yin/yang), objects that aren't completely rotationally symmetrical are quite suitable as well.

c) The attachment of the flexible connector to the pendulum body should be done at the upper center so that it can oscillate freely and without swaying.

d) The pendulum body should weight about 10 to 40 grams. The lighter it is, the better it will react. However, for this reason it will also be very instable in its oscillations, as well as difficult to interpret. The heavier it is, the more slowly it will react but also has the advantage of letting itself be read easily and precisely as a result. Simply try out different weights and choose the one that suits you best.

e) You should like your pendulum! This means that you should enjoy looking at it and handling it.

The conditions listed under a) to d) are basically of a mechanical-physical type. They are important so that you can work with your pendulum in a sufficiently precise and reliable way. Nevertheless, the last condition, listed under e), is the most important of them all! If your *Inner Child*, the level of your personality that has access to the subtle-energetic vibrations and translates these into the pendulum movements, doesn't like the pendulum it will usually just work with it in a reluctant and "stubborn" manner. So when se-

---

[1] The length of the connector should ultimately be based on whether you feel good about it. There is no optimal standard length for everyone.

lecting your "work tool," pay attention to whether your *Inner Child* exclaims "Oh! How beautiful!" when you handle it. For this reason, I also wouldn't necessarily want to get one through a mail-order business if I didn't have the opportunity of holding it and trying it out beforehand.

If you like building things, you can naturally also make a pendulum yourself according to your own special ideas. Particularly well-suited as a flexible connector is a necklace that isn't too thick. You should be able to hook a key ring onto the end of it so that you can push it over your thickest finger without any difficulty. You can hold your pendulum securely and comfortably in this manner. This is important since some pendulum oscillations, particularly above strong energy fields, can develop so much dynamic force that your instrument is practically torn out of your fingers if it isn't well attached-attached there. On the other end of the necklace, hook on another, much smaller, key ring. Then, for example, look around in stores that have crystal pendants to see if you find a small quartz-crystal tip or something similar that you would like to have as the pendulum body for your instrument. You can naturally also acquire a number of pendulum bodies for different purposes and hook them onto the key ring according to which application you want to use them for. If you would like to work with pendulum tables, for example, it's useful to have a pendulum body with a tip so that you can get precise information. However, if you "just" want to determine an oscillation pattern, you generally won't need a tip and can also use other forms of crystal.

If you would like to have a metal object as a pendulum body, the sawed-off tip of a thick carpenter's nail, through which you should drill a hole at the upper end so you can hook on the smaller key ring. You can naturally also have a piece of any sort of metal made according to your ideas for a pendulum body on a lathe in a plumber's workshop. Although this costs a bit of money, it's generally affordable and you will then have a pendulum body that truly corresponds to your own wishes.

After some time, you will probably have the same experience as almost all the passionate pendulum-users I know: you will have a constantly growing collection of all kinds of pendulums at home because time and again you find a beautiful new one that you could actually use, and even if it's just to look at. Precisely this is the *Inner Child's* play instinct!

HOW YOU SHOULD HOLD A PENDULUM

This is quite simple: A pendulum should be held in such a way that it can swing freely and not be obstructed. It also shouldn't fly out of your hand when you hold it over a strong energy field. According to my experience, the idea that a special hand position is required in order to use the pendulum in a good way and without influencing is pure fabrication. However, those who have limited themselves with such an opinion will naturally have the corresponding reactions. So don't limit yourself to this and you will have more freedom in working with the pendulum.

BASIC CONDITIONS FOR SUCCESSFUL USE OF THE PENDULUM

Things are similar regarding the basic conditions. It's not necessary to orient yourself towards a certain direction or do special exercises beforehand or only use a table without metal parts as support for the pendulum tables. Your body and your *Inner Child* are flexible, so be flexible as well and don't make life hard for them with some sort of dogma. However, work with the pendulum generally turns out better if you aren't too stressed, overtired, or too strongly emotionally moved by the topic at hand. In addition, you should free yourself as much as possible from preconceived opinions and take to heart a few basic rules for your mental attitude while using the pendulum, which I will explain in more detail at the end of this chapter.

USING THE PENDULUM AND THE THREE LEVELS OF THE PERSONALITY

I would like to go into more detail about the meaning of the three essential levels of the personality and what they have to do with using the pendulum. I call these three areas:

a) the *Inner Child*, b) the *Middle Self*, and c) the *Higher Self*. Unfortunately, there is some confusion in relation to these terms today and this is why I'm attempting to bring some order to the chaos. If you have a better understanding of these three levels of the personality, you can also more easily explain to yourself what functions and how it functions when you work with the pendulum and what doesn't work.

The *Inner Child* is a partial area of the human personality that is very much at home in the magical-mystical world of subtle energies. Through special senses that work in this area, it has a direct link to the "rest of the world," to the incarnated and non-incarnated beings, plants, animals, minerals (which are also very much alive in their own way, although modern science doesn't know anything about it yet!), and naturally to other people. For many centuries, these senses have been increasingly ignored in our latitudes and even systematically suppressed. We just have to think of the "witch"-hunting organized by the Christian churches, which lasted even up into the 19th century. This is why we practically have no words today to express the feelings that these senses impart to us. We usually ignore their messages in any case since they appear to be "illogical" and correspond too little to our "modern" view of life. This is even correct: the senses function illogically, their way of working isn't analytical but synthetic. They don't separate the world into tiny little individual pieces without any correlation but leave it as it is, namely, whole! Our *Inner Child* gets along very well with this view of the world since it's structured in precisely the same way. Just our poor intellect, which is located in another part of the personality, the *Middle Self*, has its problems with this. As a counterpoint and complement to the *Inner Child*, it has a strong analytical orientation. To put it into simple terms: the *Inner Child* is delighted when there is vanilla ice cream with raspberries and eats the whole thing with a feeling of well-being, if it feels like having it! The intellect, as an outstanding component of the *Middle Self*, first wants to know of which ingredients the food is actually composed and whether some well-known scientist holds the opinion that this would be beneficial for a person's health. If this is the case, the person dominated by the *Middle Self* would then even choke down the ice cream if it almost made him sick since it's commonly said to be healthy, he thinks.

What! You're familiar with this type of behavior? Well, no wonder since most people today have their behavior determined by the *Middle Self* here in the so-called civilized nations. This is why, in contrast to the native peoples, who are more strongly influenced by the *Inner Child*, we also have such a hard time with using the pendulum. We must learn to accept the *Inner Child*'s view of the world and way of life, at least now and then, in order to be able to further develop our subtle senses since this part of our being has sensory access to the subtle energies and not the *Middle Self*, which we are usually well-acquainted with and can also accept. The *Inner Child* then has an intensive sensory connection to the subtle levels of being. Consequently, the sensations that are translated through the muscles into the pendulum movement come through the *Inner Child's* senses. For our purposes, it's now important to take a closer look at how and in which way information is passed on to the *Middle Self*.

The *Inner Child* of a human being perceives many impressions from the subtle world through its senses. This doesn't mean it perceives all of them, as it frequently claimed, since every person is imperfect. However, each of us has a different "blind spot," so that we can complement each other well if we can accept our own imperfection. The same also applies to the "normal" senses, one person can see better than the other in relation to colors, for example. He can differentiate between the finest nuances that another person can no longer perceive. Someone else can't use her eyes as well but is capable of recognizing the components of a perfume by the smell. Furthermore, certain perceptions are emphasized in all of the senses because someone pays particular attention to them and suppresses other senses because his concentration is elsewhere. During an art exhibit, try questioning a number of people as to what they have seen and each of them will at least give you somewhat different information. Each of them has just focussed the emphasis of his attention on another theme. The last and most important thing here is: Even if two people perceive the same thing, they will still interpret it differently. According to the personal prejudices and interests, fears and desires, ideas and knowledge, maturity of character, background of experience, etc., each person will have a somewhat different opinion about the same theater performance, the same book, etc. This is why theater critics so seldom agree with each other. I've taken these examples from everyday life because we're all quite familiar with them and can talk about them. We have terms for them that everyone is familiar with.

In the world of subtle energies, which is perceived by the *Inner Child* with its keen senses, things are at least just as diversified as in the "touchable" world with which you are more familiar, but we have no generally understandable terms for them and tend to assume a skeptical attitude towards the perceptions of our senses in this regard.

For these reasons, there are two essential consequences for your involvement with the pendulum:

1) You are not and will never be infallible in the use of the pendulum![1]
2) The more tolerant, open, and attentive you are and the better you know your own talents in using the pendulum and your "blind spot," meaning the topics in which you frequently make mistakes when using the pendulum, the more securely and precisely you will be able to work with it.

There is also a third level of the personality that I haven't mentioned up to now: the *Higher Self*. Today many people claim that they have a direct line to it and their information is always correct as a result. In my opinion, such a claim is quite presumptuous and I would also like to tell you how I come up with this value judgement: the *Higher Self* is the authority within a person that watches over the fulfillment of the life plan. It makes sure that you have the experiences related to the themes in your life that you chose before your present incarnation, which we could call a type of curriculum. This plan doesn't register when and how you have an experience. These privileges remain the right of each individual as a gift of God. But whenever you evade important learning processes for a longer period of time, your *Higher Self* uses "coincidences" to suggest a few new themes. If you make use of these opportunities in due time, everything will be all right. But if you are stubborn, the hints will become more severe, up to the point of all the possible strokes of fate. It's true that your *Higher Self* is pleased to help you, should you reach and understand it, in recognizing your tasks and sometimes also gives you important hints. However, its scope of duties doesn't include clearing the problems out of the way for you or for other people. It has frequently caused them itself so that you finally wake up,

---

[1] By the way, this realization is quite widespread among well-reputed people who work with the pendulum. No true professional would claim that he or she is always right. Truly talented and experienced pendulum-users come up with a score of about 90%, with a lot of training!

pull yourself together, have certain experiences, and therefore receive the opportunity of learning and improving your personality. It also isn't interested in constantly keeping you happy and satisfied, although it doesn't have anything against you being this way as long as you learn. Whether you need this gemstone or that gemstone also isn't part of its scope of duties, the *Inner Child* with its wishes of life and its direct relationship to the material level is responsible for such things. The role that the *Higher Self* plays in using the pendulum is then conceivably minor in general. Furthermore, only the *Inner Child* can make contact with it since the *Middle Self* isn't structured holistically and can't even understand what the *Higher Self* has to tell it for this reason, we can say that the *Inner Child* interprets, and the *Middle Self* is lacking in the subtly oriented senses needed to reach the *Higher Self*. However, all the information that the *Inner Child* receives and passes on to the *Middle Self* is subject to the limitations described above, sometimes in the reception and then also in the transmission of the information (also see the related illustration on the previous page).

People generally only achieve a "standing line" to their *Higher Self* when their *Middle Self* and their *Inner Child* have matured to the extent that they shape many areas of their life out of love, the energy of unity, and not on the basis of claims to power or fear. Then they will no longer need a pendulum for the contact. However, what frequently happens is that a person's *Inner Child* wants to please the *Middle Self* and play-acts an extremely impressive *Higher Self* that presents all the possible "words of wisdom," corresponding as far as possible with the *Middle Self*'s claims to power, prejudices, and desires. It likes to be praised and loves pleasant games. If you don't want to end up in this trap, don't get insist on contact with your *Higher Self*. Be very (!) skeptical with respect to it. It's better to first work extensively on the harmonization and growth of your *Middle Self* and your *Inner Child*. Then everything else happens practically on its own. Oh, yes, one more tip: oracles that are determined by coincidence like I Ching, Tarot, Runes, Cards

PROCESSING SUBTLE PERCEPTIONS THROUGH THE INNER CHILD FOR THE MIDDLE SELF

Subtle perceptions

Inner Child

Filter
Comparison with prejudices,
fears, and memories

Question
Is the Middle Self too busy to feel its way into this?/
Does it permit the establishment of the ability to vibrate?

Question
Is there a possibility for the Middle Self
to understandably depict the subtle perception?

Information reaches the conscious mind

Most subtle perceptions are withheld through this process

Input
Possibilities of
perception/
senses

Input
Possibilities of
expression and
manipulation

Higher Self
Level of relative unity
of time and space
Tasks: Supervision of life
plan/Advice for life in holistic
sense/function of spiritual
healer/inner healer in holistic
sense

Direct perception
of all levels of
existence

"Coincidences,"
oracle
determined by
coincidence

Middle Self
Level of analysis/
material world
Tasks area: Solution of
problems in "here and now."
Rational understanding and
manipulation of the world
Setting goal for the future
and understanding the past.
Constructive realization of
emotional energies.
Creation of unconscious
patterns of thinking and
acting to facilitate shaping
of life.

All "normal
senses" like
sight, hearing,
smell, touch,
kinesthetic
sense

Language,
conscious physical
expression that is
created by physical
expression through
unconscious
pattern of thinking
and acting

Inner Child
Level of synthesis/
magic/mysticism
Task area: Acquiring power
for contact with Creation on
material level and being
willing to use it to shape your
life. Storing memories/letting
feelings flow as the
necessary synthetic
complement to the
judgments of the analytic
mind. Inner healer and
teacher in the magical-
shamanic sense.

The so-called
subtle energetic
senses: telepathy,
emotional
telepathy,
clairvoyance and
clairsentience,
precognition, the
use of the
pendulum,
retrocognition, the
ability to see auras,
and many other
types of energy
perception.

Magical-energetic
manipulations like
psychokinesis,
sympathetic magic,
transmission of
psychologically
effective energies.
Teleportation,
levitation,
materialization, etc.
Physical
expression of
emotional
energies.

of Power, etc., are directed by your *Higher Self.* When you ask precise questions, you will receive exact answers. I hope that you interpret and understand them from the proper perspective (see above). This type of perception work represents a good and, in my opinion, necessary complement to the work with the pendulum.

Taking Care of Your Pendulum

A pendulum also requires care for it to function in a reliable way. Don't worry, this isn't all that complicated. It mainly involves just three simple points:

1. You should energetically cleanse your pendulum, under cold water, for example, because it can strongly charge itself with outside energies during the work. This can obstruct its ability to oscillate on the one hand, and many outside energies can be transmitted to you and cause you to have feelings of ill-health. You can check to see whether it's "clean" by using a second pendulum.
2. You shouldn't loan your pendulum to anyone else, particularly not to people who you don't like. Your instrument functions best when it is adjusted to your own vibrations. If you do loan it to someone else, cleanse it thoroughly and then hold it for about five minutes on your HARA (a place that's located about three fingers below your navel at the center line of your body). This is the center of your personality energy, and your pendulum will attune itself to your vibrations once again through the close contact with it.
3. Keep your pendulum in a place that is peaceful in terms of its energy such as where a ficus benjamini plant[1] also thrives well. Your favorite meditation spot, a quartz-crystal geode, or a correctly built and properly oriented pyramid are well-suited for this purpose.

---

[1] A plant that reacts very sensitively to imbalanced energies.

THE BASIC PRINCIPLES
OF SUCCESSFULLY USING
THE PENDULUM

The most important principle: Never believe that you are infallible! Never use the pendulum for moral issues, for selfish reasons, for "ultimate" answers, or for information about future events. The pendulum is a wonderful instrument for the promotion of consciousness and development of the subtle senses. It isn't an oracle that has the appropriate answer to everything!

Never use the pendulum in order to find something out about another person unless you have his express permission to do so.

Always use the pendulum when you have the desire to do so and in no case when you feel an aversion against it!

Carefully verify every result, sometimes with the Error Table and further by comparing it with your knowledge, and naturally with your healthy common sense. Although the latter two aren't infallible, they can still often help you discover errors through their important commentaries.

Go ahead and thank your *Inner Child* frequently for its help and don't scold it when false results occur. Instead, talk to it about the matter, try to understand its reasons for the incorrect information, and help it (and thereby yourself) to have the courage to say the truth next time. There is a description of how to get into a conversation with the *Inner Child* in Chapter 2.

Never use the pendulum for questions that make a strong emotional impression on you or for people or about topics that you don't like. Never let yourself be put under the pressure of time or success when using the pendulum. Use a pendulum that you like and think is beautiful.

Always use your pendulum based on a feeling of deep gratitude for this wonderful gift and let the love of the entire Creation determine how you work with it.

Delusions of grandeur, fear, greed, stress, imbalances, and exhaustion will reduce your ability to use the pendulum. Modesty, gratitude, love, experiences that have been worked through, tolerance, and naturalness will certainly have a positive effect on your ability to use the pendulum, as well as on the spiritual growth of your personality.

CHAPTER 2

THE FIRST STEPS

This chapter deals with having your first practical experiences with the pendulum. In addition, on the basis of the many exercises you can already get an impression of which topics are particularly well-suited for you to use the pendulum on and where you have difficulties. Exact insight in about your "blind spot" is quite important in order to work confidently with the pendulum. It isn't important to work your way through the exercises from the first to the last. Simply try out what appeals to you. You work together with your *Inner Child* when using the pendulum, and it likes to play and performs best when doing so. This means that it focuses on fun and games instead of discipline and staying power. It may sound strange to you, but you will give yourself a great gift if you try to learn and achieve something in this relaxing and human way.

Before you start with the exercises, please read the respective instructions and follow them exactly. For various tests within one exercise, always use the same hand for the pendulum since the right and the left hand represent different polarities of the physical energy. If you change in the middle, the exact reverse oscillation of the pendulum is probable. Although you can get used to it, we want to keep the basic conditions as simple and certain as possible at the moment so that you can learn more easily. Should you wear a quartz watch, please remove it while using the pendulum. Because of the electromagnetic field that it emanates, it causes a great deal of confusion within your body and thereby impedes the translation of your subtle senses' perceptions into the movements of the pendulum. The same also applies, although to a lesser extent, to all closed metal cycles that you may possibly wear on your body in the form of rings, necklaces, bracelets, etc. Also remove them for the exercises. Later, when you have more experience, you can take the time to try out whether the jewelry disrupts or whether you can also use the pendulum with certainty when you wear it. For each experiment, have a piece of paper and a pencil ready in case you should make a note of something.

So, and now we can finally get started:

SOME SIMPLE EXERCISES WITH THE PENDULUM

Exercise 1: We can call this a warm-up exercise. Get yourself a glass of water, a gemstone, a piece of jewelry, a cup of coffee, a comic book, a novel, a spiritual book that very much interests you at the moment, and an apple. Sit down comfortably on a chair in front of a table, place the individual objects in front of you one after the other, then hold your pendulum over them and let it swing freely. Observe the various oscillation patterns.

Exercise 2: Here you can determine what language your pendulum would like to speak with you and what each movement of the pendulum means. Agree with your *Inner Child* to have oscillations that are as clear as possible. Particularly suitable are: circle to the right, circle to the left, an oscillation that is perpendicular to you, an oscillation that is horizontal to you, pendulum standstill, diagonally from you to the right, and diagonally from you to the left.

Now close your eyes for a moment, relax, listen to your breathing, and feel your body in all its areas. When you feel calm and pleasantly relaxed after a while, then focus your attention on your inner eye. Now say aloud: "I would like to have contact with you, my Inner Child. Please give me a sign of your attention." Now pay careful attention to see if there is a special perception. It may be some sort of picture, but also be a word, a sentence, a smell, or a physical sensation. When you have relaxed in advance, your *Inner*

Child will always react to your desire for contact. However, it's important that you don't overlook its perhaps quite cautious sign or dismiss it as irrelevant. As soon as you recognize its response on the basis of a certain sign, thank it for its willingness to listen to you and explain to it that you would like to learn to work with the pendulum and need its help in doing so. Ask it to translate its perceptions into pendulum oscillations so that you can understand them and promise it that you will only use the pendulum for the good of all participants and from a place of love. Moreover, tell it that it should give you a clear sign if it doesn't feel like using the pendulum for some reason. Promise that you won't pressure it in this case. Request it to tell you any possible reservations it may have at the appropriate time so that you can come to an agreement. Ask whether it now has possible reservations about cooperating with you. Pay attention to the images and/or words that describe these and try to understand them. Take the fears and desires of your *Inner Child* seriously and comply with them. Try to clarify its reservations. If necessary, find compromises that both of you can accept. However, in no case should you con your *Inner Child*. Should you have great difficulties in communicating, use an oracle like the I Ching or the Tarot. When nothing more stands in the way of an understanding, describe the possible pendulum oscillations (see above) and ask it to tell you which oscillation means what in the following exercise. Then pick up your pendulum and ask aloud: "Please show me which oscillation should mean "yes"! Wait until a distinct oscillation occurs and note this on the following table.

THE PERSONAL LANGUAGE OF YOUR PENDULUM

YOUR NAME: **DATE:**

Yes	
No	
I don't want to work on this now	
No information possible	
Affinity	
Aversion	
Yin	
Yang	
Positive	
Negative	
Neutral	
Error	

Then, one after the other, ask about the respective oscillation for "No," "I don't want to work on this now," "No information possible," "Affinity," "Aversion," "Yin," "Yang," "Positive," "Negative," "Neutral," and "Error." There will naturally be some multiple assignments, but since they can be clearly interpreted on the basis of the respective topic and the question that you have asked, it doesn't matter. It's quite possible that the assignments may change from time to time. For this reason, every few weeks you should check to see whether everything is still correct and note possible changes. As previously mentioned, children like to play and don't always like the same rules and basic conditions when doing so. Play along, nobody will become bored this way and using the pendulum will work even better! Learn the assignments by heart. This will help you work with speed and certainly at all times.

Exercise 3: This is a simple method of determining whether you need a certain energy and how much of it you need. Prepare a number of different gemstones (for example: quartz crystal, rose quartz, amethyst, agate, citrine, moon stone). Sit on a chair in front of a table. Then place one of the stones on it about 20 centimeters from the place where you hold your hand to use the pendulum. Close your eyes for a moment and relax by listening to your breathing, for example. At the close of the relaxation exercise, visualize an equilateral cross. While doing so, say out loud: "Without prejudices, I open myself up to all perceptions and request the answer to my questions, if this is right in the sense of the cosmos." Open your eyes again and now pick up the pendulum. Hold it between yourself and the crystal. Observe whether it performs an affinity, an aversion, or a neutral oscillation. In case an affinity oscillation doesn't occur, take another stone and try it once again until your pendulum shows you an oscillation of affinity. You need the energy of this stone. Put the pendulum aside and take the stone between your hands. Close your eyes and perceive its presence. Sense what's going on within your body and feel how the stone's energy does you good. When you get the feeling of having accepted enough of its energy, carry out the affinity/aversion experiment described above one more time. If an oscillation of affinity occurs again, pick up the crystal once more in order to absorb its vibrations through your hand reflex zones. When you've had enough, check it again with the pendulum. Should you get the feeling of having a certain preference or becoming tense, repeat the relaxation exercise described above, visualize the cross, and speak the related sentence in order to once again take on a neutral mental attitude. When you've received enough of the stone's energy, thank it for its gift and try out the other stones. However, you shouldn't absorb the energy from more than three or four crystals without taking a "break for digestion." When you work with large healing stones, a single stone will frequently be enough as well. Such an intensive contact often sets a great deal into motion. Your body, as well as your mind, needs time to process the energy. You can work with the pendulum in this case as well: ask it occasionally whether you should continue to work or whether it's better to take a break. Phrase the question something like: "Should I continue to work with the crystals?" Orient yourself on the information since your *Inner Child* will otherwise think that it's useless to give you advice and may possibly, at least in certain areas, discontinue cooperating with you.

Exercise 4: Plants are nice companions in life, in my opinion. But, despite loving care, some of them become stunted. In such cases, the pendulum can often help you.

Experiment a): If you have a number of potted plants standing next to each other, try holding the pendulum between two of them at a time and observe whether an oscillation of affinity or aversion results. In the latter case, it would be best for you to separate the two and bring them together with plant partners that they immediately find to be likeable. They will then grow much better and will also be less subject to attacks by pests.

Experiment b): It may also be that the energy of the location weakens the plant. This can easily be determined with your pendulum. Hold it above the plant and let it swing. If a positive oscillation results, it will be thriving quite well. If the movement of the pendulum indicates a negative oscillation, try putting it in another place and check to see whether it does better there. I have to make special mention of two phenomena that may occur since it's not all that easily to interpret them correctly. If your pendulum shows a completely strong, positive oscillation,[1] you should also move the plant to another place. Too much of a good thing can also be unhealthy. In this special case, the plant would most likely become damaged because of growing too rapidly. On the other hand, it can be totally beneficial for the health of a plant with too little vital energy to stand on a strongly positive zone for a few days in order to recharge itself. In such a case, if possible you should check every day to see whether the plant has already reached a normal energy level so that it doesn't become overcharged. At some places, the pendulum will indicate a completely balanced energy, which means that it oscillates neither positively nor negatively. Although this quality of the energy of a location is rare, it's important to know how to deal with it. Plants shouldn't constantly stand on such places. A few days or weeks are all right—but not always. This energy quality simply provides too little stimulation. The plant would be bored over a longer period of time and also become stunted. On the other hand, your green friends can take a rest here on a strongly positive place when they are exhausted from too much growth or when they have been sick and need to recuperate. For you, an energetically neutral spot is a good place for meditation and for relaxation and energy exercises.

---

[1] You have already agreed with your Inner Child in Exercise 2 as to which oscillations indicate a positive energy. You can determine the strength of the energy by the scope and speed of the pendulum's swing.

Exercise 5: Things will now get geometric! Take a piece of paper and draw lines, triangles, squares, and figures with even more corners, circles, ellipses, crosses, and an infinity sign (an eight on its side). Hold your pendulum over this page, request your *Inner Child* to show you the energy flow of the individual symbols, and see how your pendulum swings above each of them separately. In this way, you have a possibility of comprehending the energetic currents in buildings practically in a "pocket-size" format. Each symbol has a certain vibration. The master architects who built the churches in days of old knew this, as well as the creators of the megaliths, those cyclopic stone monuments from ages long past that can still be found everywhere in the world today. You can also try out an interesting application of this symbol energy for mosquito bites: draw an infinity sign (an eight on its side) with a kajal pencil, on a bite, for example, making sure that both circles of the eight are equally large. In most cases, the infection treated in this way will heal in an astoundingly short time and cause much fewer complaints.

Exercise 6: You can test the quality and suitability of drinks and foods with this method! One after the other, hold your pendulum above a piece of chocolate, a glass of pop, a fresh apple, a white-flour roll, a piece of whole-wheat bread, a fresh cucumber, a glass of tap water, and a glass of water from a medicinal spring (the water shouldn't come from a plastic bottle!). Ask your *Inner Child* to show you the vital energy in each sample through the intensity of the pendulum oscillation. Then hold the pendulum above each food and observe what happens. In this way, in the future you can quickly determine what is truly "high-quality" and what isn't. In addition, you can also hold the pendulum between yourself and the respective sample to test whether you will be strengthened (affinity oscillation) or weakened (aversion oscillation) by this food. With a little practice, you can become your own best "diet cook" in this way. The next time you cook, use the pendulum to test the strength of the vital energy in the ingredients and the finished meal afterwards. Then you will understand why you often feel so tired after enjoying food that has been cooked or fried for a long time!

Here is a further experiment with food: Determine the strength of the ready-cooked meal's vital energy with the pendulum, then say aloud: "Heavenly Father, please bless this food!" You will most likely experience quite a surprise.

Exercise 7: The pendulum can also be a big help to you when it comes to reading. What, you think you do just fine reading on your own? Well, I'll believe you this time! But maybe you'd like to try out the following experiment: Give thought to a question about a personal problem and write it down. Then pick up your pendulum and take it to your bookcase[1], hold it in front of each shelf, and ask aloud: "Is there a book on this shelf in which I can find an answer to my question?"

If your instrument shows a "no," then go on to the next shelf until it shows you a "yes." Now tap the index finger of your left hand on the back of a book and ask: "Will I find an answer to my question in this book?" If "no," then ask about the next book. If "yes," take the book out of the bookcase, open it to the table of contents and tap the first caption with your index finger. Repeat your question and turn to the corresponding chapter when the answer is "yes." Now ask about each page in accordance with the pattern with which your are now familiar. When you get a "yes," read the page and let yourself be amazed!

---

[1] I assume here that you have a bookcase, if not, then you have to go to a friend who has one. But explain your plans to him beforehand so that he doesn't call the emergency physician when you start!

Problems at the Start

There are two problems that can make it difficult for you to use the pendulum: First, it may be (rare!) that even after the exercises described above, nothing moves, your pendulum stands still and acts as if it didn't know a thing about its possibilities. Secondly, it may be that it frequently gives you the wrong answers to your questions, even if you have followed the instructions precisely. Both problems can be helped, and you will find some suggestions for this purpose in the last section of this chapter. They always work since every person, even you, has been in possession of the senses and abilities necessary for using the pendulum since his birth, whether he currently uses them or not! However, success doesn't necessarily happen from one moment to the next. Sometimes a bit of patience and more profound work is required on your part in order to (better) use your abilities. But it's worth it!

When The Pendulum Doesn't Move

First check your mental attitude towards the pendulum. Why do you actually want to use the pendulum? If you primarily want to learn this to become rich, powerful, respected, or successful, your *Inner Child* won't play along in the long run.

In this case, you should become aware of the fears that are always concealed behind such goals as the motivation and try to resolve them. If the fears are rooted deeply within you and very stubborn, I recommend that you do a series of sessions with a trustworthy therapist. It's usually much easier to resolve such fears when there are two people working together than when you try to do it as a lone fighter.

Sometimes the goal of discovering a source of infallible information is why the pendulum doesn't move. Your *Inner Child* feels rightfully overtaxed and refuses to cooperate for this reason. If you accept that every human being makes errors as long as he or she lives and is loveable particularly for this reason, this block in your ability to work with the pendulum will dissolve. Further obstacles can be stress, being overtired, or having inner tensions. Relaxation exercises like autogenic training, progressive relaxation, breathing exercises, Reiki, or similar methods can help you here. Practically every adult evening school center offers the respective classes, with the exception of Reiki, in which you can securely and quickly learn to relax. Relaxation of the body and the mind are an essential key to activating the subtle senses.

Here are a few more tips as additional help: Practice using the pendulum with things that intensely interest you, which fascinate you and make you curious. Make friends with your *Inner Child* by more frequently doing things that you simply find to be fun. In order to once again allow pendulum oscillation or strength very weak swings, an open(!) ring of copper is often helpful when placed on the small finger of the left hand. However, in some cases it works better on the right hand. Try it out! An even, gentle massage of both small fingers, particularly in the upper half, is also suitable for awakening and strengthening the ability to use the pendulum. Exercises for harmonizing the second, fourth, and fifth chakras, as well as increasing consciousness about the areas of your life organized by these energy centers, has often also cured "hopeless" cases and awakened impressive abilities to work with the pendulum.

One last important tip: If nothing else helps, get a chain or string and a pendulum body made of an *antiallergic* material like surgical steel. I was quite surprised at first when a girlfriend gave me this tip, but afterwards it became completely obvious to me. Pendulums made of antiallergic material have been able to cure some "difficult cases" up to now. Go ahead and try it out yourself!

How You Can Correct Faulty Information Given by Your Pendulum

Here as well, the first measure should be to examine your predominant motivation for using the pendulum at this time. Moreover, clarify whether the topics to be worked through make a strong emotional impression on you. Do they cause you to feel fear, greed, aversion, etc.? If this is the case, wait until you can deal with things in a more balanced way or let an uninvolved colleague work on the matter.

Topics that you should in no case work through with the pendulum are: predictions for the future, lottery numbers, stock rates, odds in games of chance and the like, contacts with the dead, with beings from "other worlds" (channeling), possession, statements about people who haven't expressly asked you to do this, statements about life and death, about past lives, karmic correlations and burdens, ultimate goals in life, as well as moral valuations of all types. These topics are not suitable for being worked on with the pendulum! I have experienced a great many people who have greatly ruined their access to subtle energies through these types of goals.

Instead, emphasize trust-building measures for your *Inner Child* and take it seriously. Respect its reservations and treat it fairly. Don't have a grim approach to the pendulum, put the emphasis on having fun! Use your mind and your intuition in a way that gives them equal rights, based on the love of the Creation, and without losing yourself in the "helper syndrome." Then your subtle senses will develop automatically and you will bring much joy for yourself and others into this world.

OPENING YOUR SUBTLE SENSES

During my involvement with the subtle senses, I have discovered a magic formula and have had it confirmed by other people time and again. This magic formula can lead anyone to an increasingly higher degree of sensitivity in the energetic realm: it is the harmonization of long-lasting disharmonious states like repulsion, competitive thinking, envy, revenge, fear, hate, blame, black-and-white thinking, embitterment, enmity, anger, arrogance, thirst for power, jealousy, frustration, not being able to let go, mistrust, rejection of one's own physical nature, pedantry, and pettiness. Each of us collects many of these energies in the course of our lifetime and doesn't let go of much of them, even to the point of making a downright cult out of them. If you accept these energies as belonging to you and learn to love yourself in a way that allows you to be/gives you the possibility of being this way, then you can integrate and harmonize them. The shadows dissolve and are transformed into radiant light. You become a bit more whole. Then you have once again decided on the path of healing love and unity, and against the dead-end street of separation. At the same time, consciously accepting the unity of all life creates more access to the senses with which you can perceive the energies of unity in your surroundings, and this then automatically intensifies and expands your ability to work with the pendulum as well.

CHAPTER 3

WORKING WITH THE READY-MADE PENDULUM TABLES

For the daily work with the pendulum, it's very practical to have an extensive collection of ready-made pendulum tables available. You'll save yourself a great deal of work and effort in drawing new ones. Now there are several things that you must take into consideration when using these tables. First, be sure that the tables you want to use also fit in with the topics to be worked on and are adequate when it comes to the number of alternatives. If there aren't enough choices available, make one yourself to which you can add the further possibilities until the topic is adequately covered in your opinion.

You can find suggestions for making your own tables in Chapter 4. Then start with the pendulum over the tables that basically treat the topic to be worked on (selection tables) in order to obtain a preselection. For example: Which therapy (Bach Flowers, biochemistry, energy work, etc.) can I use to heal a certain problem. If your instrument shows an error, then first use the Error Table in order to find out where there's a problem at the moment. In no case should you just ignore the "error" response, even if it totally annoys you! If there's no error, or if you have already successfully eliminated it, then let your pendulum show you the appropriate decision-making table, by means of which you can then come up with a concrete result. For example: Your pendulum tells you that you can find the most suitable thing in the"Biochemical Supplements" table and in working with this table you get "Magnesium phosphoricum" as the appropriate remedy. When you have reached a result in this way, hold the pendulum above the Error Table one more time to be certain. Should an error be indicated, then absolutely clarify it before you continue. Never scold your *Inner Child* because of a wrong result but always try to be open to its reservations or suggestions and come to a constructive solution that is accepted by the *Middle Self* (simplified: intellect) and the *Inner Child* (simplified: feelings). If no error is shown, inform yourself extensively about the alternative selected by your pendulum in order to examine it with your common sense to see whether it would be useful to take this path. With this process, be critical about your intellect, as well as about the information given by your pendulum. This procedure may appear to be complicated to you but, in my experience, it's the only possibility of becoming truly successful in working with this instrument. Your *Inner Child* and your intellect (*Middle Self*) must practically learn to train, understand, and accept each other so that the work with the pendulum can function optimally. Collecting knowledge about the help that the pendulum has recommended for you also brings more awareness into your life.

How often have I already had an AHA experience when my pendulum recommended a certain Bach Flower, for example, and I then read a pertinent description of my momentary psychological and energetic situation in a good book on the topic. As a result, I was capable of also supporting the healing with my intellect and more quickly recognizing the imbalanced states in the future, already dissolving them as they were first occurring. Go ahead and give yourself a chance to bring together your *Inner Child* and your intellect in this ultimately rather simple manner. One further advantage of this procedure is that extensive knowledge about a topic helps you in using the ready-made tables and creating your own in a quicker and better way.

If, for example, you are familiar with the topic of "Homeopathy" only from the captions of the pendulum tables, you will not become particularly professional in the selection and application of homeopathic remedies. You can't simply discover everything about such a topic with the pendulum! As an example of this, alone the naturally rather limited selection that you have to make for a table from the thousands of individual homeopathic remedies and combination preparations for a certain purpose (for example: healing digestive complaints) is quite difficult (to put it into mild terms) in this area without extensive knowledge. With time you will also continually expand the areas in which you can work with the pendulum and achieve an especially high degree of success, which means you can work increasingly better with it.

HOW TO USE THEM

Before you start using the pendulum, you should remove quartz watches and jewelry so that the translation of the messages from your *Inner Child* through the musculature into the pendulum oscillations won't be disrupted. Otherwise, please also think of the suggestions listed in Chapter 1 for successfully working with the pendulum. For the confident use of a pendulum table, please pay attention to the following: Hold your pendulum in the marked center of the table. Then ask your question aloud or in your mind: "Which of the alternatives available on this table can help me further in respect to ....(fill in your question)?"

If your pendulum should stand still or show the alternative "Error," use the Error Table. If you are working for someone else, be sure you have a photo of him beforehand, along with his complete first and last name, date of birth, and questions in writing that he has clearly formulated and would like to have answered. Before the beginning of the session, once again read his statements, briefly touch the photo of the respective person with your pendulum, and request helpful information for him aloud or in your mind.

Particularly for tables with many alternatives, which are located close to each other as a result, definitely use a rotationally symmetrical pendulum with a point on the lower end so that you can exactly read what your instrument would like to tell you. Be sure that you don't read the oscillation from the false perspective. Always look to see what the pendulum is doing from a position above the central point of the table. If you observe it from the side, a false interpretation could easily occur, above all in the extensive tables. Your perspective lets you see things differently than they are. After you have received an answer, you should in any case once again request a further alternative as a supplement to the first. For example, a number of Bach Flowers are put together into a mixture in order to promote healing an area of the special imbalance as extensively as possible. Only when your pendulum gives you the agreed-upon sign for "No further answers" should you end the work with this table. Each bit of information should be checked individually and all of it should be checked together at the end with the Error Table.

POSSIBILITIES AND LIMITATIONS

The possibilities result from your talent in selecting the appropriate tables for a topic or making a new table with meaningful alternatives to a topic. The selection on a table is naturally always limited. For this reason, you should always assume that your *Inner Child* tends to present you with an answer to your question that is the best approximation possible through the instrument of the pendulum. You usually don't have the optimal solution, particular for very extensive topics, on the table from the start. However, you can work your way increasingly closer to an optimal solution through the direction shown by the pendulum and the expansion of your own knowledge.

You will probably develop new pendulum tables time and again until you have good coverage of an area for most questions. Give yourself enough time in doing this and work carefully. It's always worth it! At the start of your "career" in using the pendulum, try out as many areas as possible and you can then discover what suits you best. In the course of time you can concentrate on a few areas in which you are really at home. This is a true recipe for success since you can optimally develop your abilities with the pendulum in this way.

If you become involved with too many areas in the long term, this will ultimately be at the cost of the quality. This doesn't mean it wouldn't be useful to include a new topic in your work now and then. After all, your *Inner Child* does like to play! But you shouldn't dissipate your energies in the process.

CHAPTER 4

DEVELOPING YOUR OWN PENDULUM TABLES

At some point, the ready-made pendulum tables won't be adequate for you because you are involved with topics for which there aren't any tables or for which the existing ones don't appear to be sufficient. In order to make it easier for you to make your own tables, I will give you some tips in this chapter. There are definitely a few things that you should take into consideration so that you can truly work confidently with the tables and have good results.

In addition, at the end of this book, you will find a number of sample forms to copy and enlarge to standard paper size. You can then fill them in according to the requirements of the respective topic.

DESIGNING AN APPROPRIATE PENDULUM TABLE

At the beginning of the whole action, you should make a list of all the alternatives. When you have written down all the selection possibilities, check carefully to see whether they really include everything that's necessary and nothing that's superfluous. Then draw a circle of about one centimeter diameter in the middle of the pendulum table. This is the center of the pendulum tables and the pendulum is to be positioned above it when you ask a question. You should also be above this point with your eyes so that you can properly interpret the oscillations of the pendulum. Now please count the listed alternatives and add one more to them for the information of "Error," which must absolutely be on every table. There shouldn't be more than about 43 possibilities on one pendulum table with standard paper size. Otherwise, the distances between the individual lines will be too small to read it precisely. If you need more selection criteria, then it's better to make one or more additional tables. You can then create a cross-connection to the other tables of this group on each of the tables so that the pendulum can show you where you can get suitable information if it isn't indicated on the page you're using at the moment.

If you need more selection criteria, then it's better to make one or more additional tables. You can then create a cross-connection to the other tables of this group on each of the tables so that the pendulum can show you where you can get suitable information if it isn't indicated on the page you're using at the moment. However, you can also use a pendulum table in tabular form, as described at the end of this chapter.

If you receive an uneven number of decision-making possibilities, everything is all right, but if there is an even number of alternatives, you must add a further "Error" line. Why? When there is an even number of lines that are grouped around the middle circle at the same angular distances, all the lines will be across from each other and when you work with the tables you'll never know exactly which of the two alternatives facing each other is meant. If you have an uneven number of lines that are arranged around the center in the same angular distances, this isn't a problem. The lines can face each other because of geometric reasons. Now you have to do a bit of math: divide 360 (a complete circle can be divided into 360 degrees) by the (uneven) number of lines. The number that you have come up with as a result will give you the distance in the angular degrees from one line to the next. With this as a basis, you only need to mark off the distances with a drawing triangle or another suitable protractor, draw the lines, and record the name of the corresponding alternative at their ends. If there isn't enough space to label the lines, you could also number the alternatives and just write the figure on the corresponding line. A list with the corresponding assignments should then be included in the foot text of the pendulum table. It's best to write the name of the pendulum table at the top of the page in big letters. In addition, you can note the date when you made the table in the foot text, as well as literature references on the topic worked on and, if available, the names of the other tables that belong to the group. Sometimes, for more complicated areas, it's also worth it to add a few working instructions to refresh the memory. This is particularly helpful if you don't work with this table very often.

For example, you can write down that when looking for a homeopathic remedy, you should first determined the remedy's group (such as mineral, plant, animal, element, nosode). Next, find the suitable remedy itself; then the appropriate type of potency (LM, C, X); follow this with the level of potency (such as X6). Furthermore, find out how much and how often it should be taken, as well as at what intervals. In closing, make a note to the effect of checking in a good book on pharmacology to see whether the selected remedy is appropriate and can be sensibly used in the determined dosage and type of application.

When the pendulum table is finished, you can glue it to a piece of solid cardboard that isn't too thick, punch holes at the edge, and file it into a folder. If you want to make a great many of pendulum tables, I recommend that you set up an index on the tables you have with a short description on each topic and labelling the tables belonging to a specific group at the beginning of the notebook. Although you may think that this is too complicated, it makes it much easier to do the work and helps you save a lot of time. I set up an organizing system because I found it annoying to first spend a hours collecting my pendulum tables from all corners of my home whenever I wanted to work on an interesting topic, only to discover that the most important table had been used by my cats as a substitute for the scratching post for a longer period of time. Since then, the cats haven't suffered as much from low-flying slippers and my nerves are also doing much better! If you really want to perfect your notebook, you can glue a small pocket for one of your pendulums to the inside of the cover, for example. You can also store a pencil for notes and add some empty pages at the start. Here you can jot down the results of your work, literature references, or things like supplementary exercises, the date and name of the person for whom you have used the pendulum. Then you just need to take the notebook from the shelf and you can get started. Orderliness is difficult for me as well, but believe someone who's been afflicted by chaos: It often pays off!

TABULAR PENDULUM TABLES

If you want to put a very large number of selection possibilities on a pendulum table, there is also the alternative of the tabular pendulum table. This can be structured in the following manner: draw a row of lines and columns with a pen until you have made enough squares for your selection possiblities. Now number the squares sequentially, starting at the top, from 1 to ... Then write a Roman numeral on the upper line above each column and a letter of the alphabet in the left column for each line. Write a key below the table or, according to its size, on a separate page. Here you can write the meaning of each number on the table. If you want to use the pendulum to ask about something, hold your pendulum above each column and then above each line until it starts swinging. You will find a number where the lines run together and its meaning in your key. As an alternative, you can also draw a starting point above the tabular pendulum table, from which lines run to each column. In the exact same way, put a starting point on the left side next to the table, from which lines are drawn to each line of the table. Now hold your pendulum above both of the two starting points, one after the other. Ask your question and observe which line or column it swings towards. At the point where the columns and lines cross you will again find a number, then look up its meaning in the key. To make this easier to understand, I have included a sample of a tabular table on this page (above). This type of pendulum table has two advantages: when there are a great many selection possibilities—more than 43—you still don't need more than one table. You can easily put far more than 100 alternatives on it. In addition, your intellect has less opportunity to interfere than on the normal pendulum tables because it simply loses track of things when there are so many selection possibilities and numbers given.

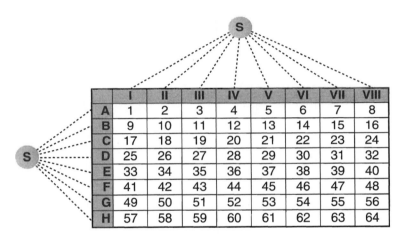

	I	II	III	IV	V	VI	VII	VIII
A	1	2	3	4	5	6	7	8
B	9	10	11	12	13	14	15	16
C	17	18	19	20	21	22	23	24
D	25	26	27	28	29	30	31	32
E	33	34	35	36	37	38	39	40
F	41	42	43	44	45	46	47	48
G	49	50	51	52	53	54	55	56
H	57	58	59	60	61	62	63	64

Example for a Tabular Pendulum Table (S = starting point)

USING THE PENDULUM IN ACCORDANCE WITH THE CHINESE FIVE-ELEMENT SYSTEM

If you frequently carry a pendulum around with you in order to always have it on hand when there's something interesting to look into, you will probably be frequently annoyed that you can't take your pendulum tables along as well. The "normal" information of "yin" or "yang," "affinity" or "aversion," "yes" or "no," isn't adequate to more closely investigate a topic on the spot. I had this feeling some time ago and, as a result, have developed a simple method that makes it possible to get extensive information about something without tables. This method uses the pendulum in accordance with the Chinese five-element system. It's an ancient system and is applied today mainly in the diagnosis and therapy with acupuncture, acupressure, and related methods. Many exercises and explanations in Tao Yoga are also based upon it. This system is particularly suited for the exploration of energetic phenomena without further background material because for generations it has contained an abundance of classifications, which have been examined time and again, that are extensive and specific enough to be capable of defining the energetic effect of a healing stone has on you at a certain point in time, for example.

However, you do need one bit of assistance in order to use this system of working with the pendulum: a small disk upon on which a circle has been drawn and divided into five fields and labelled. To make the work somewhat easier for you, such a circle is illustrated in the original size at the end of this chapter. Please copy it, glue it to a piece of solid cardboard, and color the five fields according to the terms stated there. Simply leave the white field as it is. Then copy the previous page with the classification of the five elements, which are found one page before the five-element circle, and glue this page to the back side of the cardboard. The cardboard should be large enough for all the necessary information and still fit into your pocket. Then you can always take it with you whenever you pocket your pendulum. Now you have everything you need, and we can start with the experiments.

The table is used in the following way: If, for example, you want to know the qualities of any type of healing stone at this moment—in relation to you—at a certain place[1], first touch the stone to be studied with the pendulum, then hold it above the center point of the five-element table, and ask aloud or in your thoughts: "What effect does this stone have in the here and now on me? Note the element shown and then ask about additional, weaker influences. In this way you can get quite a clear picture of the healing stone's effect on you. As an indication of an error, you can make an agreement with your *Inner Child* to use the "pendulum standing still" since the extra field to indicate this is lacking. Then you can look up the equivalents to the elements indicated and select those that fit in with the questions you want to ask. If you want to use the pendulum for someone else, also briefly tap the respective person with your instrument before starting the experiment in order to create an energetic connection. Then the matter is actually quite simple. Try out this system and experiment with it. You'll be surprised at the many interesting discoveries! It's useful to take along a little notebook and something to write with so that you can take notes in order to evaluate them later. One example: A certain power place usually has different effects on you in a certain rhythm that repeats itself at vari-

---

[1] Please absolutely(!) pay attention to this aspect when interpreting. There are hardly two people who react to the same energetic stimulation in exactly the same way. Even within the very same person, the reaction circumstances can change according to the choice of point in time and the corresponding energy of a place!

ous times. It's worth discovering these conditions because you can then work more meaningfully with the energy of that place. The energetic effect that certain people have on you can also be easily determined in this way. All you need to do this is a photo. When you've gathered some experience, you can even try out whether you can establish an adequate connection in a purely mental manner, which means that you imagine the person. This procedure is called "making mental use of the pendulum." When you try out this method, you should examine the results in a particularly thorough way until you are really sure of it. Even then, I recommend that you keep doing spot checks afterwards.

Here are some explanations about this system: It consists of the energetic elements *metal, water, wood, fire,* and *earth.*

Metal means the function of accepting and giving, communication, the metabolism, and the rhythm of life on the material and energetic level.

Water means the function of the vital and emotional energy. Everything that flows in the body, such as the lymph, blood, saliva, urine, etc., has a relationship to this element. It imparts flexibility to the body-mind-soul and the ability to let energy flow.

Wood represents growth, as well as secure rooting in the material world (grounding), and the ability to shape one's own life in a way that is responsible and meets needs. This element has a particular relationship to the spinal column and the joints.

Fire means the function of vital energy, warmheartedness, and dynamic force. Even in the Western concept of alchemy's comparable process of separating the "pure from the impure," *fire* also separates things within the body-mind-soul. It can also be symbolically described as the energy of illumination. The fire of love, sexuality, eroticism, bodily warmth, and the immune system are also controlled by the *fire* element.

Earth describes the life-bearing function of the body-mind-soul. All other energetic elements are dependent on

CLASSIFICATIONS OF THE FIVE ELEMENTS

ELEMENT:	METAL	WATER	WOOD	FIRE	EARTH
Meridians	Lungs/large intestine	Kidneys/ bladder	Liver/ gallbladder	Heart/ small intestine	Spleen/pan- creas, stomach
Sensory organs	Nose	Ear	Eyes	Tongue	Mouth/lips
Bodily components	Mucous membranes, skin	Bones	Tendons, nails	Blood, sweat	Muscles
Harmonious feelings	Courage, letting go, ability to adapt	Composure, alertness, repose	Fantasy, initiative, human warmth	Love, creativ- ity, charisma, inner strength	Inner harmony, justness
Disharmonio- us feelings	Sadness, depression	Fear, stress	Anger, hatred	Impatience, moodiness	Deliberation, worry, brooding
Sense	Smelling	Hearing	Seeing	Speaking	Tasting

PENDULUM TABLE FOR
CHINESE FIVE-ELEMENT SYSTEM

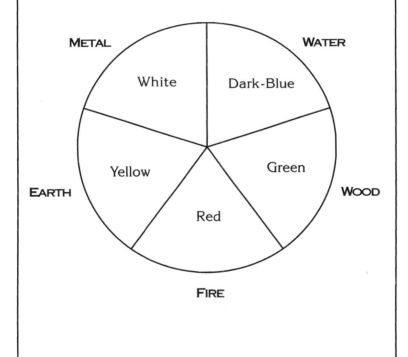

earth as a source of energy, are maintained and nourished by it. *Earthy* can also be described by the Japanese terms of "being in the *hara*," which means being centered, being at repose within yourself. *Earth* thereby lends the ability to go through the turbulent times of life and the quality of live- liness in an equilibrium and a balanced state.

CHAPTER 6

USING THE PENDULUM ON THE BODY AND PRACTICAL ENERGY WORK

Your pendulum can be a good helper for you in practical energy work for healing purposes or for spiritual development. For this reason, I will introduce some related application possibilities that I frequently use and that have proved to be quite meaningful in the practice.

MASSAGE AND PENDULUM WORK

If you would like to massage another person, both of you should first remove all jewelry and quartz watches. Now take your pendulum and position yourself about one meter from your client, face to face. Hold the pendulum in front of you and ask aloud or in your thoughts: "Which place on the body should I massage first?" If the pendulum gives you an error message, first clarify the reason behind it before you continue. If your instrument swings towards a certain area of the body, go slowly in the direction of the response until it begins to circle somewhere above the body or stands still. Now ask: "In which direction should I massage?" Take note of how it swings and then ask the question: "Should I massage with a lot of strength?" If yes, start the massage. If no, continue to ask: "Should I massage using less strength?" If yes, start. If no, ask the final question: "Should I massage very gently?" Then massage in the direction indicated and the way recommended, asking the pendulum now and then whether you should continue. When you have pampered this area of the body long enough, use the method described above to follow the pendulum in search of the next zone of the body that should now be massaged. When it no longer swings, end the session.

If there is a certain feeling of ill-health that the massage is meant to balance, ask a question that addresses the special topic at the start instead of the general question stated above. As for other applications, please remember to always check the information given for the pendulum massage. If, for example, your pendulum says you should massage your client's eyes with much pressure, you shouldn't do it—eyes are too sensitive for such experiments. When you have a quiet moment later, you should in any case clarify why your instrument has given you such a recommendation and try to eliminate the cause of the disturbance so that your abilities can be improved. In no case should you scold your *Inner Child*—it will have its reasons for such types of answers that are reasonable from its point of view. And you ultimately have your intellect in order to rule out serious errors.

AURA ENERGY WORK AND USING THE PENDULUM

Your pendulum can also help you in a similar way to dissolve energies that are stuck in the aura (aura clearing). For this purpose, I like to use crystals that have been tumbled into a round form and are about as large as a walnut. Which type of healing stone is suitable for the respective application can also be determined with the pendulum. In the appendix you will find an extensive pendulum table on the topic of "Gemstones," which is well-suited for this purpose. Once you have selected the appropriate stone, the actual work can begin.

Be sure that you and your client have taken off all jewelry and quartz watches and then stand about one-and-a-half meters away from him.[1]

---

[1] The distance is greater than for the massage this time because of the aura's diameter.

Ask your pendulum about an energy that's stuck in the aura and follow its swing until it circles or stands still. Please don't leave your pendulum at this place for very long but just for the time that's absolutely necessary in order to determine the right place—in case you haven't been initiated into a Reiki degree or don't have some other type of effective and reliable protection against the absorption of disharmonious outside energies. Otherwise, you could take on the disruptive energy yourself. Although your friend would feel better, you would feel worse and that isn't the purpose of the matter.

Then take the healing stone, which you have cleansed beforehand of outside energies with cold water or in some way that's just as good and hold it at the indicated place in the aura with three fingers. While doing this, let your pendulum swing freely and ask it to stop moving when the stone is "full." Then cleanse the stone again under cold water and bring it back to the previous position in the aura. Again ask your pendulum to oscillate until the stone is full or the disharmonious energy has been eliminated. If it stands still, ask whether the disruptive energy has been balanced. If not, cleanse the crystal again and repeat the procedure until your little helper gives you a "green light." It's totally possible that there will be a number of places in the aura with blocks. So, to be sure, always ask one more time and pay attention to whether the stone that you have been using is suitable for the dissolution of another disorder. You may sometimes need to use various stones in one session.

When the aura clearing has been completed, give your client some pure and natural (!) lavender oil and let him rub it on his main chakras, as well as the palms of the hands and soles of the feet. Then, he should rest for at least fifteen minutes. Afterwards, for several days he should continue with rubbing in the lavender in the morning after getting up. This serves to create an undisturbed restructuring and healing of the energy system. After the session, wash your hands and lower arms thoroughly with flowing water. Also cleanse the healing crystals that you've used. If you have applied some of them a number of times, you should give them a "breather" for a few days. Lay them in the sun, next to a large, strong plant, under a Reiki shower[1], or on a crystal geode so that your little friends can recuperate from the hard work. Before you go to bed at night, you should definitely shower with lukewarm(!) water in order to let go of outside energies that have possibly gotten into your aura. If at all possible, you should air the clothing that you have worn during the session outside overnight before you wear it again.

HEALING STONES AND PENDULUM WORK

The pendulum can serve you well in selecting the stones for a crystal healing. In the appendix you will find a corresponding table in case you don't want to make your own. When you have found the appropriate stone for dissolving a disharmony, you can let the pendulum show you the places on or around the body—which is also frequently the case—where the crystals should be used. In this simple manner, you can compile effective crystal healing patterns for certain problems that are optimally attuned to the respective person. Crystal patterns are many times more effective than individually applied stones or necklaces.[2]

---

[1] A Reiki shower is a stationary Reiki energy field that can be built with the possibilities of the Second Degree. It has a strong cleansing and vitalizing effect on everything that's inside of it.

[2] By the way, it's not really recommended that you constantly lug healing stones around with you in every form! Their strong energies can also produce disharmonies within the body or even intensify existing ones under certain circumstances! If the crystals aren't energetically cleansed (cold water, large crystal geode, sunlight, Reiki, etc.) on a regular basis, they can additionally radiate disharmonious energies back to the body when they are overcharged with them. As applies to all strong healing remedies, crystals should only be used with much thought and expertise.

They are, so to speak, the high art of crystal healing. The powers of the individual healing stones mutually intensify each other and also make possible the harmonization of deep, even constitutional disorders.

The development of the personality can also be freed of impasses and accelerated through the appropriate healing stone patterns. Before you use the pendulum and the crystals, both you and your client should remove jewelry and quartz watches, as usual. All stones must be carefully cleansed beforehand and afterwards (see above). In this highly effective form of crystal work, you should pay special attention to monitoring errors and inform yourself comprehensively about this area before you start working with it or with large crystals.

After an application, your client should use lavender once again, as described above, and rest for at least thirty minutes. During the next days, he should drink much clear water. Some days beforehand and afterwards, the consumption of alcohol, coffee, cigarettes, and other drugs should at least be greatly reduced. You shouldn't treat serious health disorders without professional supervision if you aren't a naturopath, psychotherapist, or doctor!

ESSENCES AND PENDULUM WORK

Essences can often be used much more successfully by rubbing them into the suitable skin zones than by just taking them orally. To my knowledge, up to now there is only a good classification of the individual body areas for the Bach Flower Essences. Your pendulum can assist you here. Position yourself about one meter away from your client, who should be lying down, and ask the pendulum about a body zone that is particularly suitable for rubbing in a certain flower essence. If you use the Bach Flower Essences, it can help you make the decision as to which zones should be treated by rubbing in a certain remedy. Never use the essences direct from the stock bottle for rubbing purposes—use only the dilutions!

The applications described in this chapter are very effective! Please use them in a responsible manner. For all serious diseases of body and mind—and for everything that could be of a more serious nature—you are both legally and morally obligated to consult a person with the suitable professional qualification (doctor, naturopath, psychotherapist) if you aren't a professional yourself!

It should be easy for you to develop your own methods on the basis of the exercises described here. You will also find many suggestions through the literature on the individual subjects in the Commented Bibliography in the appendix. Go on a journey of discovery—it's worth it!

CHAPTER 7

FINDING EARTH RAYS AND OTHER DISRUPTIVE FIELDS

Many diseases and feelings of ill-health can only be harmonized when the affected person protects himself against subtle disruptive rays or exposes himself to them to a much lesser degree. Among such harmful energies are: earth rays from faults, coal seams, water veins; the so-called Global Grid (GGN) and the Curry Grid, two systems of energy lines that circle the world with quite a high degree of symmetry in their course; the special energies of power places; rays from transformers, electric stoves, monitors (television sets), microwave ovens, and power transmission lines.

Your pendulum can help you in recognizing subtle disruptive rays so that you and others can be protected from them. However, before I go into more detail about this, I would like to give you background information on the topic of disruptive fields and disease.

Rays of all types also constantly surround us in a natural environment—which means uncultivated surroundings. Various types of cosmic rays affects us every second of our life as well. A certain "exposure to rays" is apparently a part of our natural environment. We obtain a large portion of our own vital energy through the points of the acupuncture meridians and the body's diverse main and secondary chakras from these fields. In addition, they offer us a certain "natural stress" that our body-mind-soul absolutely needs in order to train its energetic immune system and receive developmental stimulation on all levels. The situation with this energetic "stress" is quite similar to that of the material level with its bacteria, viruses, and fungus spores that occur everywhere. Our physical immune system depends on them for constant training and the continual further development of its abilities.

A person who is healthy in the holistic sense, which means someone who primarily lives in harmony with himself and the world, will not become seriously ill on the basis of this natural stimulation. They must even be present in order to guarantee his long-term well-being. A healthy person can even cope with a short-term increase of various types of rays. But the situation always become difficult when someone is either exposed to a high level of rays on a long-term basis or, for one reason or another, has a weakened vital-energy structure that can no longer adequately protect him from the normal outer influences over a longer period of time. Both of these cases are the subject of this chapter. Before you can deal with this phenomenon, it's first important for you to learn to determine the strength of a person's vital-energy field (the energetic immune system) in order to know whether he copes with the normal ray stimulation without damage to his health. On the other hand, you must train yourself to filter out the sources of rays found within the scope of a normal intensity when you go hunting with the pendulum in order to be able to find the truly stressful disruptive rays. Only then will you get results that do justice to the practice and not become confused in the jungle of many everyday rays.

DETERMINING THE STRENGTH OF THE ENERGETIC IMMUNE SYSTEM

Use the following method to determine the vital energy of a human being: turn to the page with the pendulum table "Amount of Vital Energy" in the appendix (pg. 102). Briefly touch the person whose vital energy you want to determine with your instrument in order to create an energetic connection. Now ask your *Inner Child* aloud or in your thoughts: "How high is the current vital energy of this person in percent, if 100 is his possible maximum value?" The pendulum will now show you a certain value. Continue to ask: "At which value in percent is his energy too low in order to protect him against the exposure to rays that normally occurs in his surroundings?" Now look at the new value to see whether it's lower than the first. In this case, everything is all right and you can now continue to research whether there is unusual exposure to rays in this person's life. How to do this is explained below.

However, if the new value is close the first or possibly even higher, you should be careful. In any case you should check the results in the usual way and additionally use the following method. Ask your pendulum: "Does the cause of this person's feelings of ill-health lie in an exposure to rays?" If you don't get a "yes" and there's no negative information from the Error Table when checking this, you should first thoroughly investigate to see whether there are other causes for the imbalance, even if your client still insists on "rays." If the reason for the health disorder can actually be found in the weakness of the vital energy, methods such as Bach Flower Essences, Reiki, homeopathy, gemstone therapy, or psychotherapy can contribute to a healing, depending on the type of disorder. Sometimes a change in diet is also completely adequate for this purpose. Here you can naturally also have your pendulum help you. It naturally isn't absolutely necessary to ask the pendulum in order to select a possibility for healing. If time is running short, the next obtainable and acceptable possibility should immediately be put to use. And if certain promising methods are easily available, there's absolutely no reason not to first try these out before asking the advice of the pendulum. Use this valuable helper sparingly! Although it can be used in many ways, you should in no way(!) make yourself or others dependent on it. People still have—thank God—a great many other possibilities for making a decision. The pendulum should be a helper but more of an adviser than a decision-maker, particularly in important life situations.

DIRECTLY LOCATING
DISRUPTIVE RAYS

If the too intensive effects of rays is the cause of the imbalance, you must then determine where its source is. Before you start looking, think about the following: the affected person generally won't be thrown out of his energetic balance because of "passing by" strong rays. There are a few exceptions to this, which I will discuss in greater detail at the end of this chapter.

For this reason, it's useful to investigate the places where your client frequently is and/or stays for a longer period of time for higher-than-average disruptive rays. Examples of this may be the where someone sleeps, the television armchair, or the place of work (perhaps in front of a computer?!). Make up a corresponding list with him. When doing this, pay particular attention to places that were newly added during a time period of about six months before the beginning of the affliction (change of residence, change of sleeping place, new job, or similar factors). In this way you will very quickly achieve a limitation of the possible causes. Moreover, clarify whether new electrical or sewage-related installations have been built in the direct or immediate surroundings of the places he prefers to be during this period of time.

Once you have worked out a "plan of action" in this way, you can follow it up by going to the various locations with the pendulum. In order to fade out the normal exposure to rays, you can build a kind of filter together with your *Inner Child* before the investigation. To do this, you need either the presence of your client or a photo of him, as well as a relaxation exercise: when you have arrived at the site to be investigated, close your eyes for a moment and concentrate on your breathing until you feel completely well and relaxed. Then request that in the following investigation your *Inner Child* doesn't indicate all the energy sources that are too weak to energetically harm your client. Now open your eyes once again and touch the person for whom you want to work—or a photo of him—with the instrument in order to create the necessary energetic connection. Now you can let the pendulum swing and ask it the question as to which place in this room is a harmful source of disruptive rays for your client[1].

Slowly follow its oscillation so that you can recognize deviations in the swing in due time until it clearly shows you a certain energy quality. Then determine the type and intensity of the field before you search for further "troublemakers." In order to be able to properly identify the energy quality, you should become familiar in good time with the fundamental knowledge described in the following digression and let your *Inner Child* show you a distinct type of oscillation for each of the five basic forms of rays discussed here.

If, while walking around, you receive from your pendulum indicates specific rays, it's useful to note the place, spread, and intensity of the rays for later evaluation.

You can determine the intensity by taking the table "Amount of Vital Energy" (pg. 102) that you've already used above, relaxing, and telling your *Inner Child* that you would like to know how many months your client could stay in this rays without harmful effects and that each of the 100 graduation marks should stand for one month in the process. Then, in the same way, ask about weeks, then days, then hours, etc. These statements are naturally related to the current vital-energy status of the respective person. If this changes, the tolerance values will obviously change as well!

---

[1] This classification is important! As you know from the previous chapters, the same energies have differing effects on different people.

DIGRESSION: FIVE TYPES OF DISRUPTIVE RAYS

A digression is necessary at this point so that you can recognize and interpret the various basic forms of disruptive rays. I differentiate between *yang rays*, *yin rays*, *constantly changing rays*, a *stasis field*, as well as a *ray hole*. *Yang rays* basically represents a constant flow of energy to the place located within the ray area. So-called waking zones, meaning places on which sensitive people have a hard time going to sleep, but can work well and with staying power, have a distinct yang quality. Excessive *yang rays* becomes apparent in such afflictions as nervousness, irritability, sweating, cramps, a tendency towards inflammations and high blood pressure, diarrhea, runny nose, or nausea.

Yin rays provides a constant flow of energy away from the area within the ray zone. So-called fatigue or cancer zones, meaning places at which people quickly fall into a relaxed state, tending towards weakness, have a distinct yin quality. Excessive *yin rays* can manifest themselves through such conditions as tiredness, a general feeling of exhaustion, a lack of dynamic force in the life signs, freezing, a tendency towards degenerative diseases (such as cancer), constipation, lack of appetite, blood pressure that is too low, weakness of the body's defensive systems, or circulatory disorders.

Constantly changing rays result, as the name already implies, from strong rays of various qualities. The stronger the rays are and the more frequently they change their characteristics, the more disharmonious the effect on human beings can be. The human energy system with its highly complicated and interlocked regulating mechanisms is overstrained by the constantly changing strong stimulation and reacts with disturbed functions, overreactions and underreactions, metabolic dysfunctions of all types, manic-depressive states, all possible forms of allergies, increased aggressiveness, a feeling of being overworked, immune-system weakness, migraines, a lack of zest for living, and—after a longer period of time—apathy, meaning deficient responsiveness, or exactly the opposite, hypersensitivity. I call these effects of the *constantly changing rays* the "culture syndrome."

You will find many fashionable complaints of our age in the examples listed. We live in a ray environment that's continually getting more complicated. With each new electrical device, with every further water pipe, each new stretch of directional radio, each additional radio or television transmitter, catalytic converter in a car[1], etc., the rays of the environment in the cultivated areas of our world become even more complicated and intensified.

A *stasis field* is either (usually) a zone in which various polar energy qualities do something like mutually cancel each other or (seldom) a special form of ray that has the effect of slowing down all types of vital processes. The effects are, for example, absentmindedness, a feeling of not belonging to this world, the loss of grounding, unrealistic attitudes, deficient detoxification on the organic level, an overall more sluggish metabolism, decrease in performance, and weakness. However, this is usually without degenerative cell formation. Dullness, possibly with a tendency towards stronger tension and a general lack of energy, without the health disorders that normally develop on this basis, can occur.

A *ray hole* has very distinct effects on a human being: he becomes bored. A longer stay in such an area may result in a lack of flexibility, general listlessness, and a tendency towards groundless provocation, disharmonious aggressiveness, and "snobbery." If a person isn't exposed to enough

---

[1] Catalytic converters also transmit rays into the inside of the automobile that are intense and often constantly changing in its quality. The disharmonious effects can be determined in the occupants with a pendulum after longer drives, as well as with modern measuring equipment for the various forms of vital energy. As so often, our science has given us a device that is useful on the one hand, but can also further tax our health on the other hand.

challenging stimulation, he will try to create tension situations on his own.[1]

In order to round off the picture, I would like to briefly point out the positive effects of the various energy forms. Nothing in the world has just one side to it ...

Strong *yang rays* can reactivate sluggish life functions and, for example, have a positive effect on depressive people and those who suffer from general exhaustion. Strong *yin rays* can generally bring excessive energies (for example, in the case of hysteria or inflammations) down to a tolerable level, calm fears, and generally support relaxation. Powerful, *constantly changing rays* are capable of positively influencing inflexibility on all levels, setting processes of learning and maturation into motion, creating stimulation for development, bringing forth sensitivity, promoting decision-making processes and thereby the ability to say "yes" and "no," and also uncompromisingly translate this decision into action. Now you can also explain why we shape our culture as we are currently doing. We live in an age of transition! It's necessary for the survival of humanity as a whole to develop consciousness, accept personal responsibility, and make very clear decisions for and against certain paths. Since, for reasons of economy, people can only develop when they are challenged, our *High Selves* must create the corresponding basic conditions on the threshold to the Age of Aquarius that give us learning stimulation. This is hard but heartfelt—isn't it?!

A *stasis field* promotes all types of enlightenment situations (there are a great many different expressions of this condition). This is a space without decisions and interests. In such a field, a person has the opportunity of letting his situation have its effect on him dispassionately, from a distance, and without taking sides.

---

[1] The symptoms listed here frequently occur with the given classification, but not always. In accordance with the respective person's ability to respond, the symptoms can also be manifest in a completely different way. This is why you should always precisely determine the type of disruptive rays!

But he shouldn't stay in it for too long because otherwise there's the danger of no longer knowing why he should do and not do anything at all and therefore prefer to withdraw from this place. A *ray hole* can be a good place to recuperate after many learning experiences and developmental processes. If you remember the description of the effects of the last-mentioned energy quality, you'll certainly have an easier time imagining that a longer period without stimulation can come after some further hectic years of transition if we have learned what is necessary. If we don't understand certain things, it may be that we all take the pause for rest with each other on the subtle levels. As the quintessence of this section, you should keep in mind the phrase "too much is unhealthy!".

A tip: The specified basic energies can be differentiated even further through classification with the Chinese five elements, the qualities of the meridians and main and secondary chakras that we are familiar with from acupuncture. In these classifications, please note that a *yang ray*, for example, has the quality of a certain chakra, giving it energy and virtually charging it. *Yin ray* of the same type draw energy away from this energy center. *Constantly changing rays* provide it with developmental stimulus, which it can integrate and grow through or reject and be caused to dysfunction as a result. A *stasis field* with a certain chakra quality can offer it the possibility of being without expectations and thereby opening up and becoming enlightened. A *ray hole* can provide the associated center with a breather and regeneration break after a hefty phase of development. The *possible* effects given in this example are correspondingly valid for the other areas listed above.[1] So—and now on with the practice. I hope this excursion into theory didn't bore you all too much ...

---

[1] Here as well, please remember that these classifications are usually—but not always—valid! So examine the individual cases!

Indirectly Locating Disruptive Rays

Sometimes it isn't possible to walk through the place in which your client spends his time. In such cases, you can help yourself with an indirect investigation method. However, this requires some practice in working with the pendulum if you want to get exact results. So don't start too early with it and examine what you've worked out with great care.

Have your client make you a sketch of the relevant premises, supplemented by photos of the building in which these are located, as well as the address. Then relax and in this state ask your *Inner Child* for help in the following investigation. Explain to it that the sketches represent the actual rooms and that you would like to determine the places of disruptive rays on these sketches with the pendulum. Then proceed as described above in the direct location and don't forget to also take notes here for evaluation later.

Harmonizing Earth Rays

After so much information about finding earth rays, you will certainly also want to be able to harmonize such disruptive fields. Here are a few tips on this subject:

An essential aspect, according to which you should evaluate all the direct remedial remedies, is discovering the meaning of a certain type of disruptive ray for the affected person. In other words, why has he shaped his life in such a way that he has exposed himself to such damaging rays. When you investigate the corresponding rays as to not only their fundamental quality, but also their classification to the chakras, for example, and associate this result to the life of the client, you won't be able to get over your amazement for a long time to come. People who try to sidestep certain influences in their life in order to avoid the learning process that results from confrontation with this stimulus often are ordered disruptive rays with the corresponding quality from their *Higher Self*—

quite coincidentally, of course. This portion of the body-mind-soul is responsible for the promotion of a human being's development and sometimes there's probably nothing else for it to do than resort to such drastic measure in order to finally initiate long-overdue learning steps. If you can make these correlations clear to your client, you will ultimately help him to live a much more harmonious and happy life than if you just provide him with a biofield-formation device. In plain English: if you just help him suppress the rays at the site, he will most probably have further developmental stimulation pushed at him by his *Higher Self* in some other way, which could be even more taxing. If, for any reason at all, it's too much for you to work on this, ask your client to look for an esoterically oriented personal counselor who can intuitively obtain the necessary information for him from the aura, through an oracle, or in any other way, and thereby help him find the paths of harmonious growth.

The "technical" aspect—meaning the suppression of rays—is naturally important as well. If a person is so sick that he can't even crawl, then he also has no energy to learn and grow on new paths. I can't unconditionally agree with many of the usual self-help recommendations like bowls with quartz sand, agate, or other healing stones, straw mats, millet pillows, holy water, cactus, and the like. Sometimes they help for a certain period of time, but usually they don't help or don't help enough. And crystals in particular, if they aren't selected and applied with much expertise, can cause a great deal of additional damage by focussing and thereby intensifying the disruptive rays. In addition, the personal energy of the stones can also be damaged by strong irradiation, and I think that's unfair. If it isn't possible to shift the lifestyle to another, less-radiated place as the simplest and most effective remedy, you should use the specially developed biofield-formation devices. As a supplement(!), plants of all types, rugs made of organic materials, wind chimes, etc., can be used as well.

However, there are two types of disruptive fields that you can't eliminate with a biofield-formation device. The first of these is the ray hole. In order to get help here, you must use strong plants, expressive works of art, an interior decoration with diversified colors, interesting furniture, aquariums, and the like. This will bring harmonious energies into the room lacking in energy and fill it with life. The other type of disruptive ray is the second form of the *stasis field*, meaning the independent type that hasn't been created by balancing opposing energies.

The best help here is to not expose yourself to such a field on a regular basis. The next best is to fill the room with non-polar energy (= Reiki) using the methods of Second Degree Reiki over a longer period of time until the *stasis field* is removed or get the help of an experienced Feng Shui specialist.

There is no list of companies offering biofield-formation devices in this book because of the limited space and because such a list would quickly be out-of-date.

HEALTH DISORDERS CAUSED BY SHORT-TERM EFFECTS OF RAYS

As promised above, I will go into more detail about this topic: The causes of such disorders are often x-ray examinations of very sensitive people or of those who are fasting or primarily live from a vegetarian raw-foods diet. Both of these situations can so weaken the normal energetic defence mechanism that the energy shock of an x-ray examination or related methods can drastically effect the regulatory systems of the organism. Increased radioactive values in the environment (Chernobyl, A-bomb tests, etc.) also have similar effects. A change of diet for a time and the use of appropriate homeopathic remedies, Bach Flowers, Reiki, or other suitable methods by a person with expert qualifications(!) can be excellent and provide quick help. In addition, here is a tip for the "home medicine cabinet": the consumption of organic miso, a special soybean preparation from Japan, is said to help eliminate or at least reduce the harmful effects of high level of exposure to radiation.

CHAPTER 8

THE PENDULUM TABLES

You will find an extensive collection of pendulum tables in the appendix following this chapter so that you can get involved in the practice right away. The Decision Tables are connected with each other through the respective Selection Tables that precede them in order to guarantee systematic and meaningful use in "your daily pendulum work."

HOW SHOULD YOU USE THE PENDULUM TABLES?

Here is the simplest method first: If you have a totally concrete question such as which fragrance oil you should now drip into your volitalizer in order to sweeten your work, turn immediately to the Decision Table[1] "Aromatherapy" and let yourself be shown the suitable fragrance by your pendulum.

If you would like to work on a problem for which you either aren't certain or don't know at all where to find an approach to a solution , then it's best for you to use the Selection Tables. First formulate a question. For example: "What can help me in mastering my relationship problems?" Then leaf to the first pendulum tables with the heading "Group Selection Table" and let the pendulum suggest a group of tables for you. If you land at the statement "Error Correction" with this first question, please don't skip over it

---

[1] "Decision Tables" is what I call pendulum tables that give you a series of concrete statements to make your decision easier. For example, some aromas, the main chakras, or Bach Flowers. "Selection Tables" is what I call the pendulum tables that name a series of Decision Tables, from which you can then find the most appropriate one with the help of your pendulum.

but work carefully with this table and think about the information that your pendulum comes up with. If you end up with another group, turn to the Selection Table preceding this group and let your pendulum show you the competent Decision Table. Using this, you can then find an appropriate approach to the solution.

If, at first glance, you have landed at an inappropriate group or table, don't immediately throw this information into the wastepaper basket. The pendulum often tries to tell you something indirectly in this manner that isn't indicated on the tables available for selection. In such a case, you should give considerable thought to the supposedly senseless information, feel what's going on inside yourself, meditate about it, or do something else that you think may help you to decode the hidden answer. Perhaps you would like to have your pendulum also show you an appropriate oracle on the "Oracles and Guides" table that would be particularly suitable for explaining the pendulum's response to you.

USE OF THE INDIVIDUAL PENDULUM TABLES

The pendulum tables in the appendix are very comprehensive and can be used in many ways. Particularly when you want to approach a problem area in a serious and profound way in order to find a solution for yourself or others, it's absolutely necessary for you to be extensively informed about it. This will also increase the quality of your ability to work with the pendulum. All the possible areas naturally aren't covered by the pendulum tables since there are simply too many of them to do this. So please excuse me if exactly your "specialty" isn't represented here. In case you at some time want to work in an area that isn't included or is just partially included in the tables, make your own. If you're like me and tend to read books starting at the back:

I've given an exact explanation of how you can make tables that fit your own needs in Chapter 4.

Reminder: If person is seriously ill or there's a possibility that this is the case, he must be treated by a doctor, naturo-path, or psychotherapist in accordance with the type of health disorder. If you aren't a professional, please just use the pendulum tables suitable for diagnosis and choice of therapy within the scope of a home medicine cabinet or for preventive purposes. In no case should you take on more responsibility then you can bear with a good conscience!

That's it! With all my heart, I wish you a great deal of enjoyment in working with the pendulum and much love and light on your path.

PENDULUM
TABLES

Pendulum Tables—Index

GROUP SELECTION TABLE

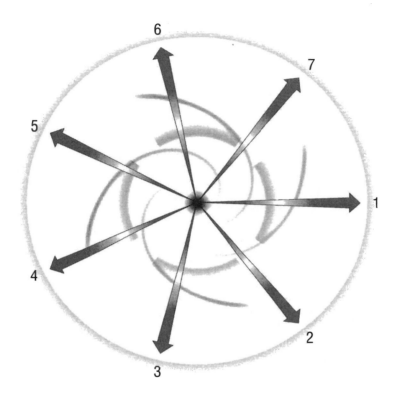

1 Error Correction, pg. 87
2 Health and Anatomy, pg. 88
3 Diet, pg. 93
4 Energy Work, pg. 103
5 Homeopathy and Essences, pg. 115
6 Spiritual Growth and Self-Knowledge, pg. 183

7 Relationships and Partner-ship, pg. 190
8 Money, Profession, and Possessions, pg. 195
9 Your Own Pendulum Table, pg. 200

ERROR CORRECTION

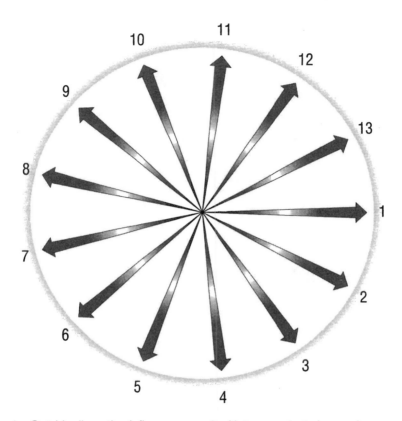

1 Outside disruptive influences
2 Lack of trust
3 Bias
4 Not seriously interested
5 Answer not on this table
6 Vanity
7 Incompetence

8 Not concentrated enough
9 Too tired
10 Disruptive magical influences
11 Respect the privacy of others
12 Not permitted to answer at
   this time
13 Error

HEALTH AND ANATOMY

SELECTION TABLE

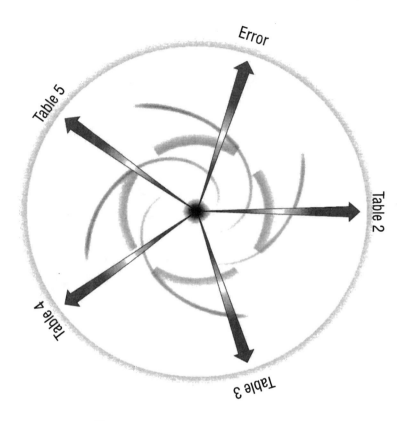

Error
Table 2—Inner Organs, pg. 89
Table 3—Glands, pg. 90
Table 4—Spinal Column, pg. 91
Table 5—Causes of Health Disorders, pg. 91

INNER ORGANS

HEALTH AND ANATOMY—TABLE 2

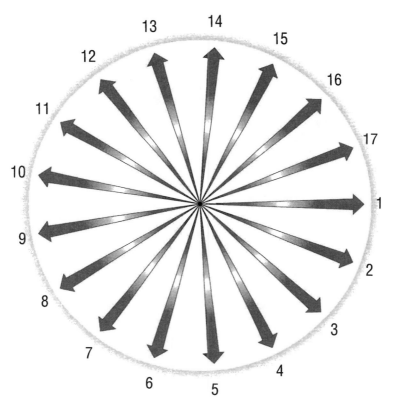

1	Brain	10	Pancreas
2	Spinal cord	11	Spleen
3	Spinal column	12	Bladder
4	Lungs	13	Sexual organs
5	Heart	14	Large intestine
6	Kidneys	15	Small intestine
7	Gallbladder	16	Duodenum
8	Bone marrow	17	Error
9	Stomach		

GLANDS

HEALTH AND ANATOMY—TABLE 3

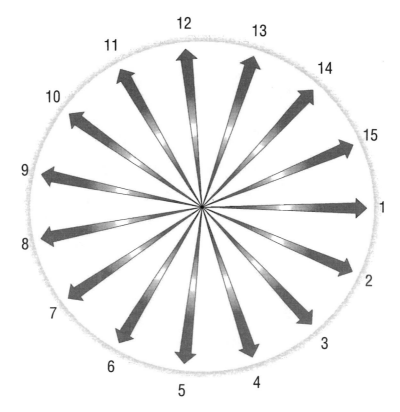

1	Stomach	9	Salivary gland
2	Intestines (excretory)	10	Thymus gland
3	Intestines (incretory)	11	Pancreas
4	Liver	12	Pineal gland
5	Thyroid gland	13	Pituitary gland
6	Parathyroid gland	14	Sexual glands
7	Adrenal gland	15	Error
8	Bronchial gland		

Spinal Column

Health and Anatomy—Table 4

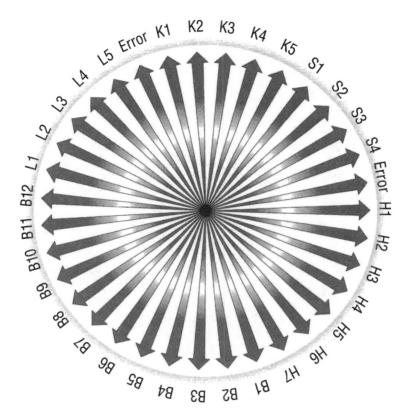

H 1-7 Cervical vertebrae 1,2,3,4,5,6,7
B 1-12 Dorsal vertebrae
       1,2,3,4,5,6,7,8,9,10,
       11,12
L 1-5 Lumbar vertebrae 1,2,3,4,5
K 1-5 Sacral vertebra 1,2,3,4,5
S 1-4 Coccygeal vertebrae 1,2,3,4
       Error

Causes of Health Disorders

Health and Anatomy—Table 5

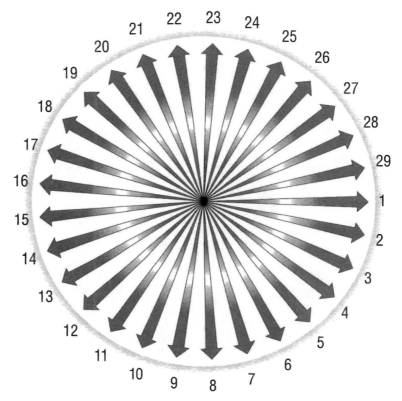

1 Earth rays	12 Insufficient demands on emotions	21 Excessive mental demands
2 Technical disruptive rays	13 Other sources of contagion	22 Excessive emotional demands
3 Scars	14 Insufficient ability to detoxify	23 Place with disharmonious energy
4 Spinal column	15 Insufficient receptivity	24 Disharmonious relationship
5 Teeth	16 Improper diet	25 Chakra block
6 Disharmonious posture	17 Radioactivity	26 Meridian block
7 Too little vital substances	18 Chronic infection	27 Possession
8 Too little water	19 Karma	28 Drugs
9 Too much water	20 Excessive physical demands	29 Error
10 Insufficient demands on body		
11 Insufficient demands on mind		

DIET

SELECTION TABLE

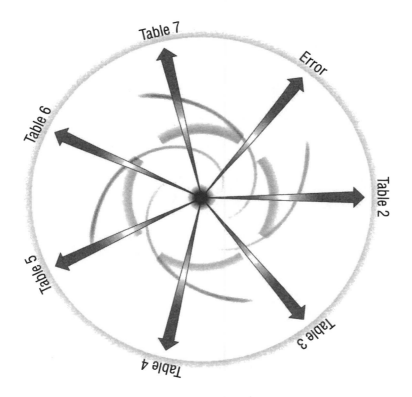

FOOD SUPPLEMENT AND VITAMINS

DIET—TABLE 2

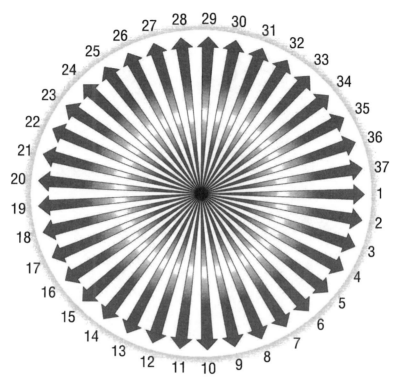

1 A	15 PABS	27 Chromium
2 D	16 C	picolinate
3 E	17 B_{13}	28 DHEA
4 K	18 B_{15}	29 Melatonin
5 B_1	19 B_{17}	30 Catuaba tea
6 B_2	20 Alpha-lipoic acid	31 Pau d'Arco tea
7 Niacin	21 Bioflavonoides	32 Enterostatyn
8 B_6	22 L-Carnitine	(kiwi pill)
9 Pantothenic acid	23 Essential fatty	33 Grapefruit seed
10 Biotin	acids	extract
11 Folic acid	24 Q 10	34 Black cumin oil
12 B_{12}	25 Lecithin	35 Essiac
13 Myo-inosite	26 Rutin	36 Guarana
14 Cholin		37 Error

MINERALS AND TRACE ELEMENTS

DIET—TABLE 3

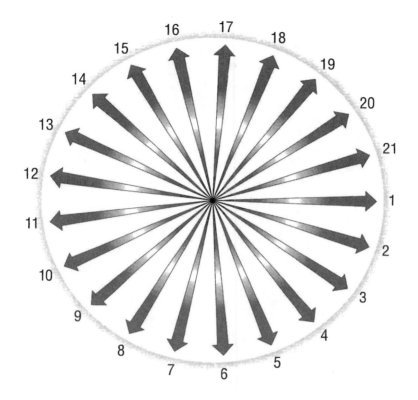

1	Iron	12	Gold
2	Fluoride	13	Lithium
3	Magnesium	14	Zinc
4	Copper	15	Nickel
5	Calcium	16	Lead
6	Potassium	17	Aluminum
7	Cobalt	18	Tin
8	Iodine	19	Manganese
9	Boron	20	Selenium
10	Silicon	21	Error
11	Silver		

VARIOUS TYPES OF DIETS

DIET—TABLE 4

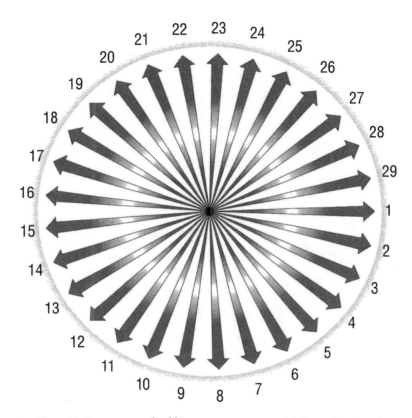

1 Macrobiotics	9 Vegan	19 Less denatured
2 Hays food	10 Mixed diet	food
combination	11 More meat	20 Fasting cure
3 Raw fruit and	12 Less meat	21 Mayr cure
vegetable diet	13 More raw fruits	22 Waerland diet
4 Fit for Life	and vegetables	23 Fresh whey cure
5 Highly nutritious	14 Less raw fruits	24 Eat more food
diet according to	and vegetables	25 Eat less food
Bruker	15 Ayurvedic diet	26 Drink more liquids
6 Intuitive diet	16 Deacidification	27 Drink less liquids
7 Hollywood Star	diet	28 Fruit cure
diet	17 Less sugar	29 Error
8 Ovo-lacto	18 Less salt	
vegetarian		

Food Components

Diet—Table 5

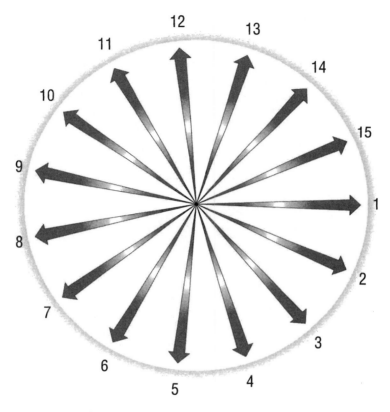

1	Proteins	8	Vital energy
2	Carbohydrates	9	Water
3	Fats	10	Chlorophyll
4	Minerals and trace elements	11	Salt
5	Vitamins	12	Acids
6	Enzymes	13	Alkalines
7	Roughage	14	Flavoring
		15	Error

IMPROVING THE ENERGETIC QUALITY OF FOOD

DIET—TABLE 6

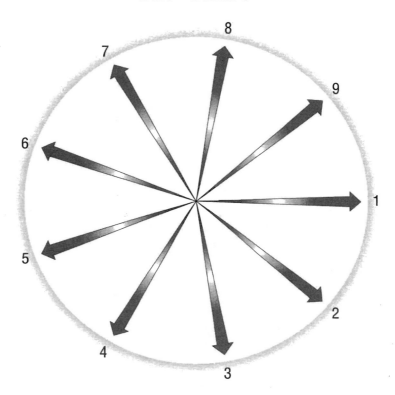

Charge with:
1 Gemstones
2 Reiki
3 Pyramid energy
4 Your own vital force

5 Color energy
6 Verana© color foils
7 Blessing
8 Giving thanks
9 Error

FOOD WITH A HIGH LEVEL OF HEALING EFFECTS

DIET—TABLE 7

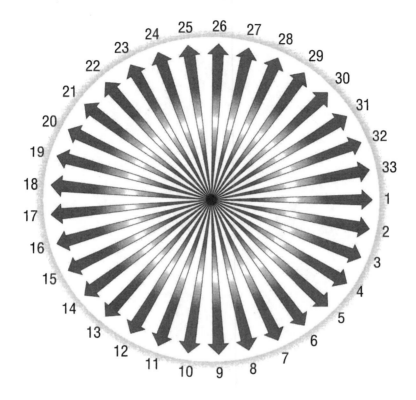

1 Ginger	13 Watermelon	25 Ghee
2 Garlic	14 Grapes	26 Miso
3 Onion	15 Bananas	27 Umeboshi plums
4 Cabbage	16 Wheat sprouts	28 Gomasio
5 Potato	17 Alfalfa	29 Boiled water
6 Topinambur	18 Prunes	30 Natural honey
7 Yam root	19 Sauerkraut	31 Mare's milk
8 Pineapple	20 Celery	32 Medicinal mineral
9 Mango	21 Green salad	water
10 Papaya	22 Dandelion	33 Error
11 Strawberries	23 Red beets	
12 Kiwi	24 Avocado	

PH-VALUE

SUPPLEMENTARY TABLE A

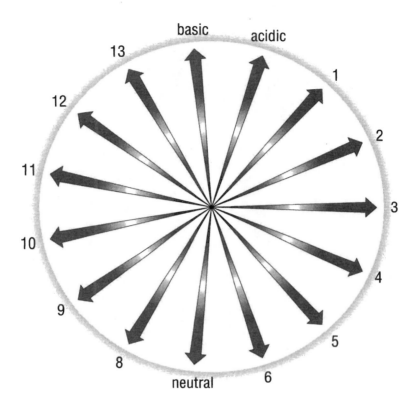

0	(acidic)	8	
1		9	
2		10	
3		11	
4		12	
5		13	
6		14	(alkaline/basic)
7	(neutral)		

Yin-Yang Relationship

Supplementary Table B

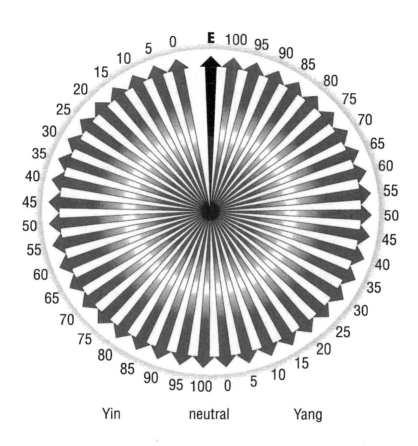

AMOUNT OF VITAL ENERGY

SUPPLEMENTARY TABLE C

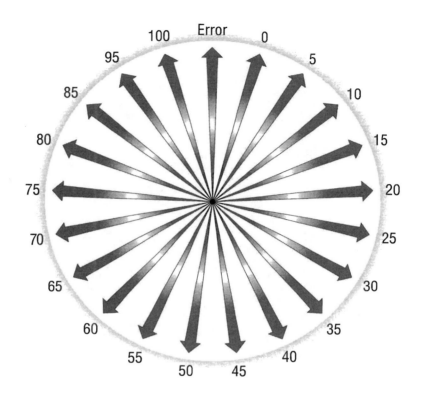

0   Minimum
100 Maximum

ENERGY WORK

SELECTION TABLE

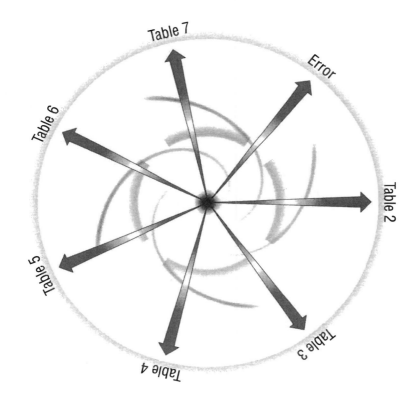

Error
Table 2—Healing Stones, pg. 104
Table 3—Aromatherapy/Oils, pg. 110
Table 4—Systems for Directing and Freeing
    Vital Energies, pg. 111
Table 5—Color Therapy, pg. 112
Table 6—Affirmation and mantras, pg. 113
Table 7—Meditation, pg. 114

HEALING STONES

ENERGY WORK—TABLE 2
Group Selection Table

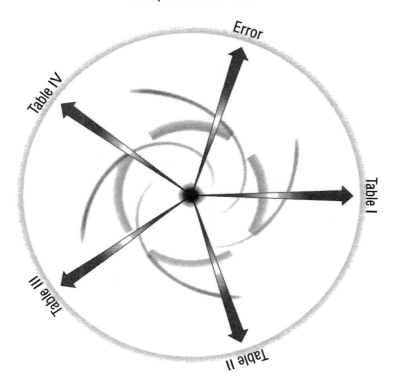

HEALING STONES TABLE I

ENERGY WORK—TABLE 2

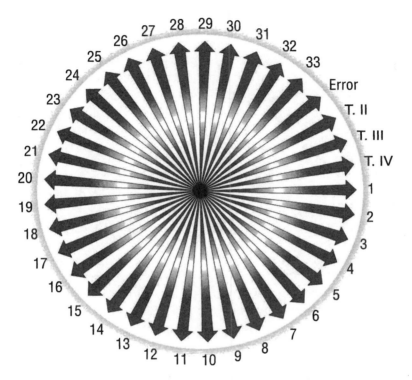

1 Actinolite	16 Boji's	28 Chrysoberyl-alexandrite
2 Agate	17 Botryoid blende	
3 Amazonite	18 Calcite	29 Chrysocolla
4 Amber	19 Carnelian	30 Chrysoprase
5 Amethyst	20 Chalcedony, blue	31 Citrine
6 Ametrine	21 Chalcedony,	32 Coral, black
7 Antimonite	copper-chalce-	33 Coral, pink
8 Apatite	dony	34 Error
9 Apophyllite	22 Chalcedony,	35 Healing Stones
10 Aquamarine	dendrite	Table II
11 Aragonite	23 Chalcedony, pink	36 Healing Stones
12 Aventurine	24 Chalcedony, red	Table III
13 Azurite	25 Charoite	37 Healing Stones
14 Azurite-malachite	26 Chiastolite	Table IV
15 Beryl	27 Chrysoberyl	

HEALING STONES TABLE II

ENERGY WORK—TABLE 2

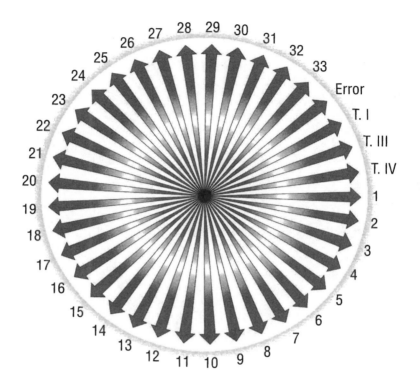

1 Coral, red	15 Garnet-hessonite	28 Lapis lazuli
2 Coral, white	16 Garnet-melanite	29 Larimar
3 Diamond	17 Garnet-pyrope	30 Lepidolite
4 Dioptase	18 Garnet-rhodolite	31 Malachite
5 Disthene-cyanite	19 Garnet-spessartine	32 Marble
6 Dolomite	20 Garnet-uvarovite	33 Moldavite
7 Dumortierite	21 Hawk's-Eye	34 Error
8 Emerald	22 Heliotrope	35 Healing Stones
9 Epidote	23 Hematite	Table I
10 Fluorite	24 Jade	36 Healing Stones
11 Garnet	25 Jasper	Table III
12 Garnet-almandine	26 Kunzite	37 Healing Stones
13 Garnet-andradite	27 Labradorite	Table IV
14 Garnet-grossulare	(spectrolite)	

HEALING STONES TABLE III

ENERGY WORK—TABLE 2

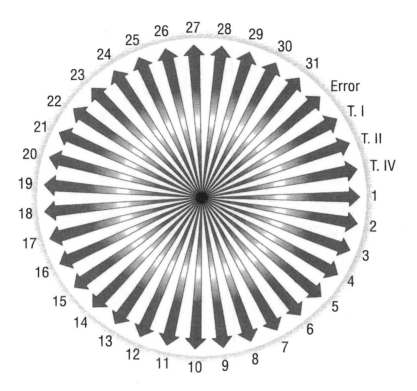

1 Mookaite	14 Peridot (olivine/ chrysolite)	26 Rose quartz
2 Moonstone	15 Pethalite	27 Ruby
3 Morganite	16 Pietersite	28 Rutile quartz
4 Moss agate	17 Porphyrite	29 Sapphire
5 Nephrite	18 Prase	30 Sardonyx
6 Obsidian	19 Phrenite	31 Serpentine
7 Onyx	20 Pyrite	32 Error
8 Opal	21 Quartz crystal	33 Healing Stones Table I
9 Opal-chrysopal	22 Realgar	34 Healing Stones Table II
10 Opal-fire opal	23 Rhodochrosite	35 Healing Stones Table IV
11 Opal, green	24 Rhodonite	
12 Opal, pink	25 Rhyolite	
13 Pearl		

Healing Stones Table IV

Energy work—Table 2

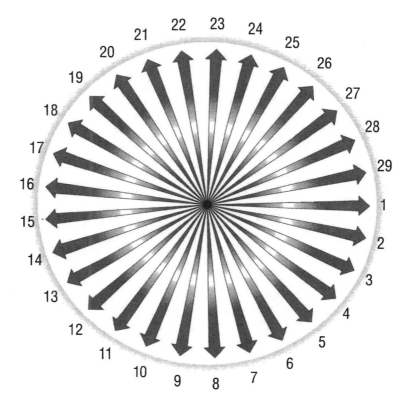

1 Smoky quartz	13 Tourmaline	20 Tourmaline-
2 Sodalite	(general)	Watermelon
3 Spectrolite	14 Tourmaline-	tourmaline
4 Staurolite	dravite	21 Tree agate
5 Sugilite (luvolite)	15 Tourmaline-	22 Turquoise
6 Sunstone	elbaite	23 Ulexite
7 Tansanite	16 Tourmaline-	24 Variscite
8 Thulite	indigolite	25 Wood, petrified
9 Tiger's-Eye	17 Tourmaline-	26 Zinc blende
10 Tiger-Iron	rubellite	27 Zircon
11 Topaz	18 Tourmaline-	28 Zoisite
12 Topaz Imperial	schorl	29 Error
(golden topaz)	19 Tourmaline-	
	verdelite	

TYPES OF APPLICATIONS

ENERGY WORK—TABLE 2
Supplementary Table A

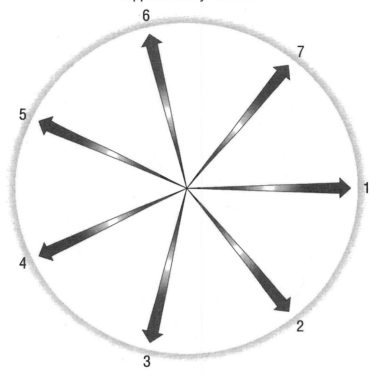

1	Place on spot	5	Wear on body
2	Gemstone meditation	6	Make contact
3	Lay out healing pattern	7	Error
4	Gemstone essence		

AROMATHERAPY/OILS

ENERGY WORK—TABLE 3

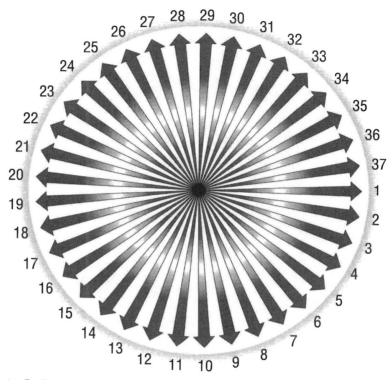

1	Basil	14	Incense	27	Patchouli
2	Benzoin	15	Jasmine	28	Pepper
3	Bergamotte	16	Juniper	29	Peppermint
4	Cajeput	17	Lavender	30	Pine
5	Camomille	18	Lemon	31	Sage
6	Caraway	19	Lemon grass	32	Sandalwood
7	Cardamom	20	Melissa	33	Sassafras
8	Cedarwood	21	Mint	34	Swiss stonepine
9	Clary sage	22	Myrrh	35	Verbena
10	Cypress	23	Neroli	36	Ylang-ylang
11	Eucalyptus	24	Orange	37	Error
12	Galbanum	25	Oregano		
13	Geranium	26	Palmarosa		

Systems for Directing and Freeing Vital Energies

Energy Work—Table 4

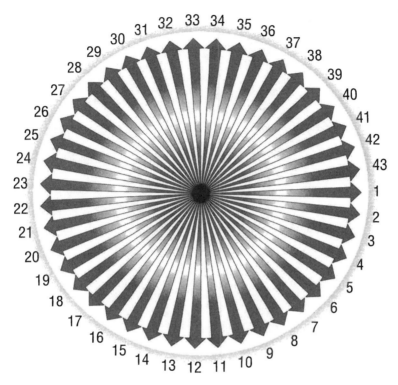

1 Acupuncture	15 Gestalt therapy	31 Rebirthing
2 Alexander technique	16 Homeopathy	32 Reichian body work
3 Analytic psycho- therapy	17 Huna	33 Reiki
4 Autogenic training	18 Hypnotherapy	34 Reincarnation therapy
5 Belly dance	19 Jin Shin Do	35 Scan therapy
6 Bioenergetics	20 Kinesiology	36 Shiatsu
7 Breathing therapy	21 Martial arts	37 Spagyric
8 Core energetics	22 Meditative painting	38 Sport
9 Eutonie	23 Metamorphic method	39 Tai Chi Chuan
10 Family therapy	24 Overtone singing	40 Tantra
11 Fasting	25 Polarity	41 Triadic therapy
12 Feldenkrais	26 Postural integration	42 Yoga
13 Fire walk	27 Primal therapy	43 Error
14 Foot-reflex zone- massage	28 Psychodrama	
	29 Qi Gong	
	30 Rebalancing	

Color Therapy

Energy Work—Table 5

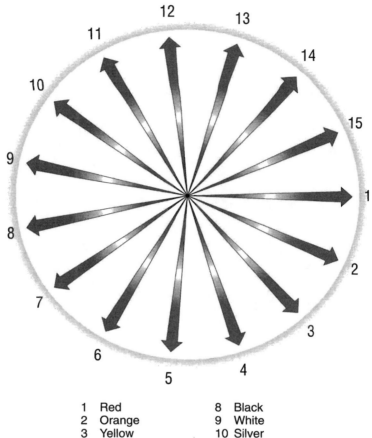

1	Red	8	Black
2	Orange	9	White
3	Yellow	10	Silver
4	Green	11	Gold
5	Blue	12	Brown
6	Indigo	13	Gray
7	Violet	14	Pink
		15	Error

112

Affirmations and Mantras

Energy Work—Table 6

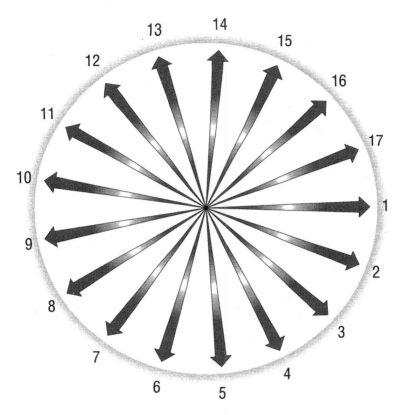

1   I love myself just as I am
2   I like to give and take
3   I am a light-filled creature of God
4   OM
5   Amen
6   Namu Amida Butsu
7   MU
8   I happily flow with the stream of life
9   I live in the here and now
10 Jesus
11 Sun
12 Moon
13 OM mani padme hum
14 OM namah shivaya
15 I am connected with everything on the deepest level
16 I receive everything that I need at the right time
17 Error

Meditation

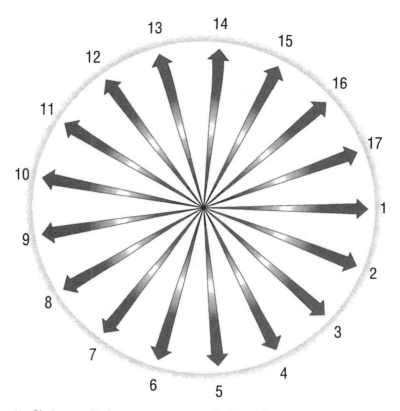

1 Chakra meditation	10 Mandala meditation
2 Three-ray meditation	11 Meridian meditation
3 Darkness meditation	12 Nadabrahma
4 Dynamic meditation	13 Rune meditation
5 Gemstone meditation	14 Transcendental meditation
6 Kirtan	15 Vipassana
7 Kundalini meditation	16 Zazen
8 Latihan	17 Error
9 Light meditation	

HOMEOPATHY AND ESSENCES

SELECTION TABLE

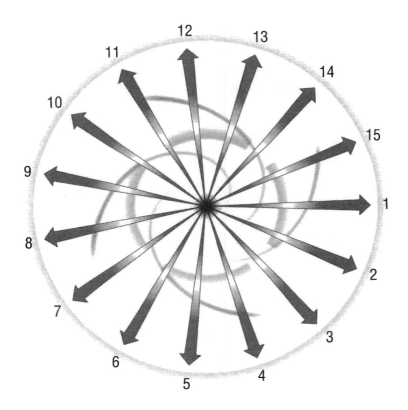

BACH FLOWERS

HOMEOPATHY AND ESSENCES—TABLE 2A

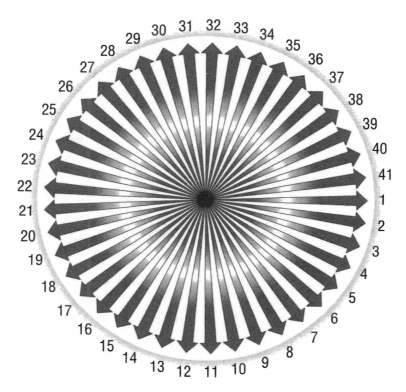

1 Rock Rose	15 Olive	29 Sweet Chestnut
2 Mimulus	16 White Chestnut	30 Star of Bethlehem
3 Cherry Plum	17 Mustard	31 Willow
4 Aspen	18 Chestnut Bud	32 Oak
5 Red Chestnut	19 Water Violet	33 Crab Apple
6 Cerato	20 Impatiens	34 Chicory
7 Scleranthus	21 Heather	35 Vervain
8 Gentian	22 Agrimony	36 Vine
9 Gorse	23 Centaury	37 Beech
10 Hornbeam	24 Walnut	38 Rock Water
11 Wild Oat	25 Holly	39 Rescue Remedy
12 Clematis	26 Larch	40 Error
13 Honeysuckle	27 Pine	
14 Wild Rose	28 Elm	

AFRICA RESEARCH ESSENCES

HOMEOPATHY AND ESSENCES—TABLE 2B

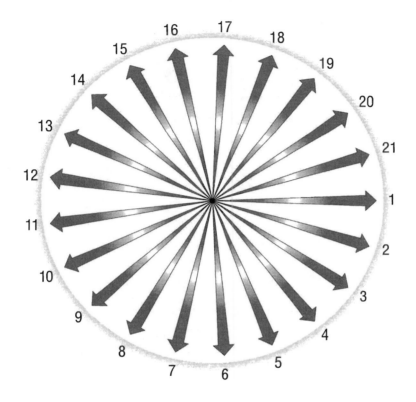

1	Banana	12	Mimosa
2	Bird-of-Paradise Flower	13	Monstera
3	Canadian Creeping Bellflower	14	Pimpernel
4	Canadian Wormwood	15	Poinsetta
5	Coconut Palm	16	Rockrose
6	Crinoline Narcissus	17	Rose Mallow
7	Echium	18	Tachinaste, White
8	Eucalyptus	19	Tree Heath
9	Geranium	20	Error
10	Leadwort	21	Error
11	Milk Thistle		

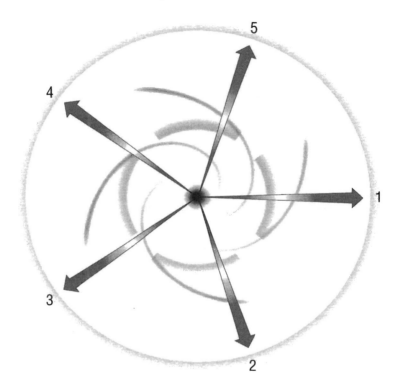

ALASKAN FLOWER ESSENCES

HOMEOPATHY AND ESSENCES—TABLE 2C

1. Topic: Becoming Clear

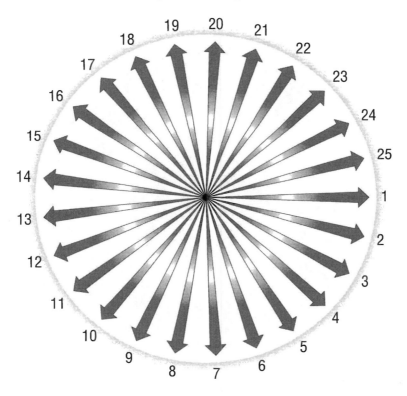

1	Alder	
2	Balsam Poplar	
3	Black Spruce	
4	Blue Elf Viola	
5	Chiming Bells	
6	Cotton Grass	
7	Dandelion	
8	Fireweed	
9	Forget-Me-Not	
10	Foxglove	
11	Golden Corydalis	
12	Green Bells of Ireland	
13	Icelandic Poppy	
14	Jacob's Ladder	
15	Labrador Tea	
16	Lady's Slipper	
17	Monkshood	
18	Paper Birch	
19	Prickly Wild Rose	
20	Spiraea	
21	Twinflower	
22	Wild Iris	
23	Willow	
24	Yarrow	
25	Error	

ALASKAN FLOWER ESSENCES

HOMEOPATHY AND ESSENCES—TABLE 2C
2. Topic: Who Am I?

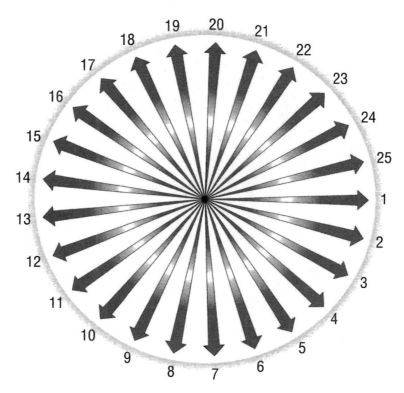

1 Alpine Azalea	10 Lace Flower	19 Tamarack
2 Bog Blueberry	11 Mountain	20 Tundra Rose
3 Bog Rosemary	Wormwood	21 Unchberry
4 Cassandra	12 Opium Poppy	22 White Spruce
5 Columbine	13 Pineapple Weed	23 White Violet
6 Cow Parsnip	14 River Beauty	24 Yellow Drias
7 Grass of Parnas-	15 Single Delight	25 Error
sus	16 Sticky Geranium	
8 Grove Sandwort	17 Sunflower	
9 Horsetail	18 Sweet Gale	

Alaskan Flower Essences

Homeopathy and Essences—Table 2C

3. Topic: Self-Realization

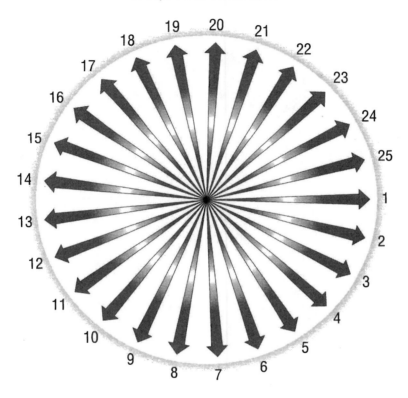

1 Attail Pollen	10 Lamb's Quarters	17 Sitka Burnet
2 Bladderwort	11 Moschatel	18 Sitka Spruce
3 Blueberry Pollen	12 Northern Ladies'	Pollen
4 Comandra	Slippers	19 Soapberry
5 Green Bog	13 Northern Twayb-	20 Spagnum Moss
Orchid	lade	21 Sweet Grass
6 Green Fairy	14 One-Sided	22 Tundra Twayb-
Orchid	Wintergreen	lade
7 Hairy Butterwort	15 Round-Leaved	23 White Fireweed
8 Harebell	Sundew	24 Wild Rhubarb
9 Ladies' Tresses	16 Shooting Star	25 Error

ALASKAN FLOWER ESSENCES

HOMEOPATHY AND ESSENCES—TABLE 2D
Environmental Essences

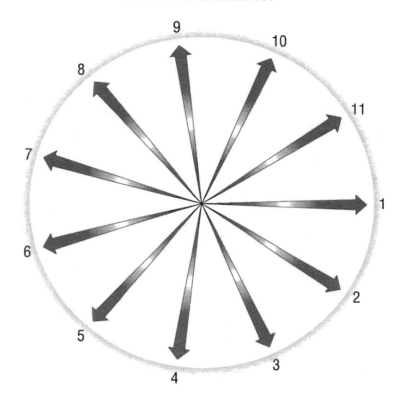

1 Chalice Well—Opening Up to the Help of the Angels
2 Full Moon Reflection—Self-Enlightenment
3 Glacier River—Letting Go of the Past
4 Greenland Icecap—Purposeful Devotion
5 Liard Hot Springs—Purification and New Creation
6 Northern Lights—Changing the Pattern in the Heart
7 Polar ICe—Patience in Times of Transition
8 Portage Glacier—Purification and New Animation
9 Rainbow Glacier—Opening Up to the Physical World
10 Solstice Storm—Letting Go and Becoming Renewed
11 Tidal Forces—Flowing with the Transition

ALOHA HAWAIIAN FLOWER ESSENCES

HOMEOPATHY AND ESSENCES—TABLE 2E
Group Selection Table

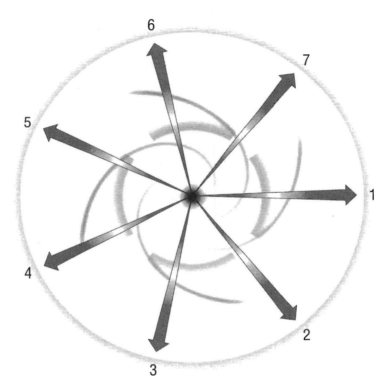

1 Sexual Identity, pg. 124
2 Support of Healing, pg. 125
3 Energetic Protection, pg. 126
4 Spiritual Development, pg. 127
5 Social Contacts, pg. 128
6 Error
7 Error

ALOHA HAWAIIAN FLOWER ESSENCES

HOMEOPATHY AND ESSENCES—TABLE 2E
1. Topic: Sexual Identity

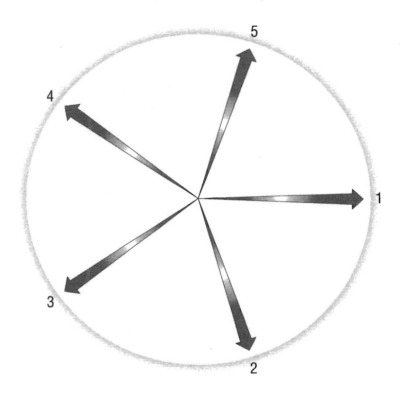

1 Lehua
2 Niu (Coconut)
3 Noni
4 Error
5 Error

ALOHA HAWAIIAN FLOWER ESSENCES

HOMEOPATHY AND ESSENCES—TABLE 2E
2. Topic: Support of Healing

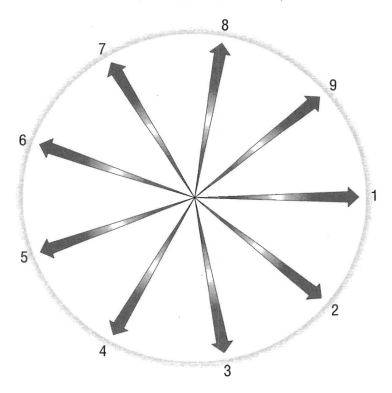

1   Coffee
2   Hawaiian Tree Essence
3   Hau
4   Ili'Ahi
5   Mango
6   Ohai Alli
7   Stock Rorrish
8   Yellow Ginger
9   Error

ALOHA HAWAIIAN FLOWER ESSENCES

HOMEOPATHY AND ESSENCES—TABLE 2E
3. Topic: Energetic Protection

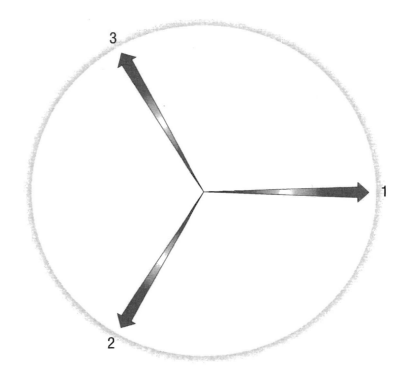

1   Ti (Ki)
2   Error
3   Error

ALOHA HAWAIIAN FLOWER ESSENCES

HOMEOPATHY AND ESSENCES—TABLE 2E
4. Topic: Spiritual Development

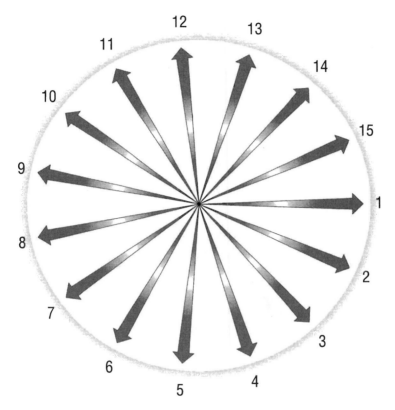

1	Angel's Trumpet	9	Ohelo
2	Avocado	10	Papaya
3	Bamboo Orchid	11	Passion Flower
4	Bougainvillea	12	Pukiawe
5	Ilima	13	Thanksgiving Cactus
6	Koa	14	Wiliwili
7	Kou	15	Error
8	Naupaka Kahakai		

ALOHA HAWAIIAN FLOWER ESSENCES

HOMEOPATHY AND ESSENCES—TABLE 2E
5. Topic: Social Contacts

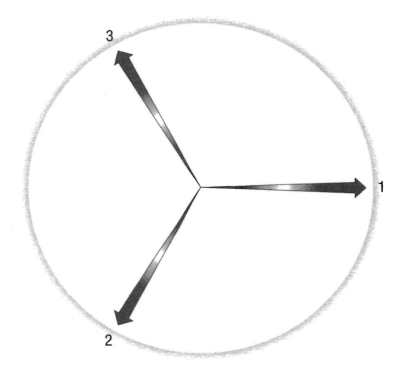

1   Kukui
2   Ulei
3   Error

AUSTRALIAN LIVING FLOWER ESSENCES

HOMEOPATHY AND ESSENCES—TABLE 2F
Group Selection Table

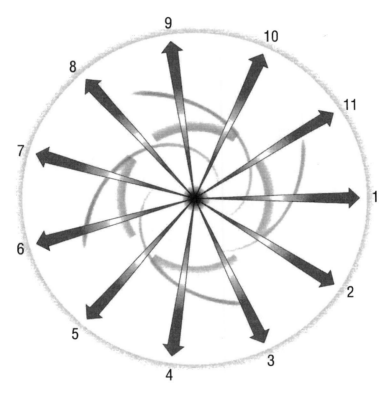

1 Healing, pg. 130
2 Letting Go, Being in the Flow,
  Letting It Happen, pg. 131
3 Harmonizing Negativity, pg. 132
4 Willingness to Love, pg. 133
5 Self-Confidence, pg. 134
6 Facing Up to Life, pg. 135
7 Spiritual Development, pg. 136
8 Vitality, Clarity, Ability to Act, pg. 137
9 Social Contacts, pg. 138
10 Error
11 Error

AUSTRALIAN LIVING FLOWER ESSENCES

HOMEOPATHY AND ESSENCES—TABLE 2F

1. Topic: Healing

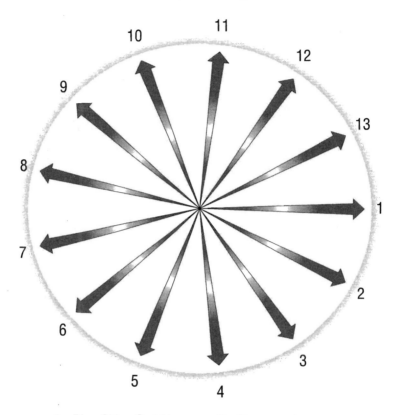

1	Blue China Orchid	7	Macrozamia
2	Cowkicks	8	Menzies Banksia
3	Fuchsia Gum	9	Pink Fairy Orchid
4	Hops Bush	10	Purple Flag Flower
5	Illyarrie	11	Star of Bethlehem
6	Kolokoltchik	12	Error
		13	Error

AUSTRALIAN LIVING FLOWER ESSENCES

HOMEOPATHY AND ESSENCES—TABLE 2F

2. Topic: Letting Go, Being in the Flow, Letting It Happen

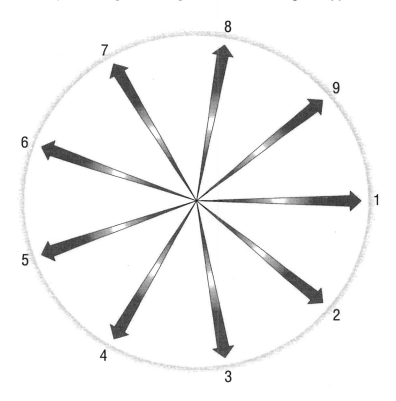

1 Brown Boronia
2 Correa
3 Dampiera
4 Golden Waitsia
5 Mauve Melaleuca
6 Red and Green
  Kangaroo Paw I
7 Russian Centaurea
8 Wild Violet
9 Error

131

AUSTRALIAN LIVING FLOWER ESSENCES

HOMEOPATHY AND ESSENCES—TABLE 2F

3. Topic: Harmonizing Negativity

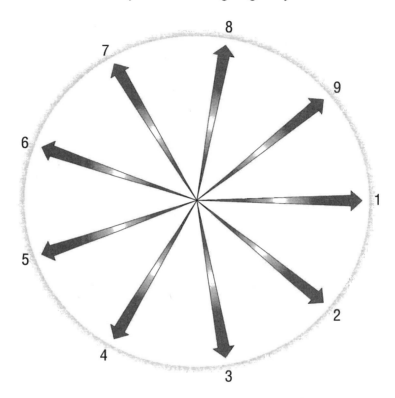

1. Fringed Lily Twiner
2. Fringed Mantis Orchid
3. Fuchsia Grevillea
4. One-Sided Bottlebrush
5. Pale Sundew
6. Purple and Red Kangaroo Paw II
7. Ribbon Pea
8. Wallflower Donkey Orchid
9. Error

AUSTRALIAN LIVING FLOWER ESSENCES

HOMEOPATHY AND ESSENCES—TABLE 2F
4. Topic: Willingness to Love

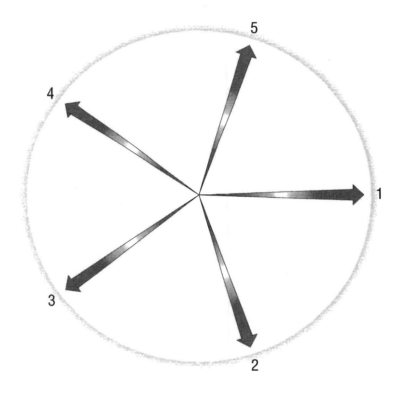

1   Black Kangaroo Paw
2   Capa Bluebell
3   Orange Leschenaultia
4   Purple Eremophila
5   Error

AUSTRALIAN LIVING FLOWER ESSENCES

HOMEOPATHY AND ESSENCES—TABLE 2F
5. Topic: Self-Confidence

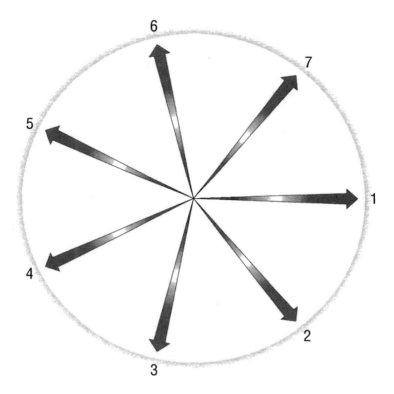

1 Happy Wanderer
2 Hybrid Pink Fairy
  Cowslip Orchid
3 Pink Impatiens
4 Russian Forget-Me-Not
5 Urchin Dryandra
6 Yellow Cone Flower
7 Error

Australian Living Flower Essences

Homeopathy and Essences—Table 2F
6. Topic: Facing Up to Life

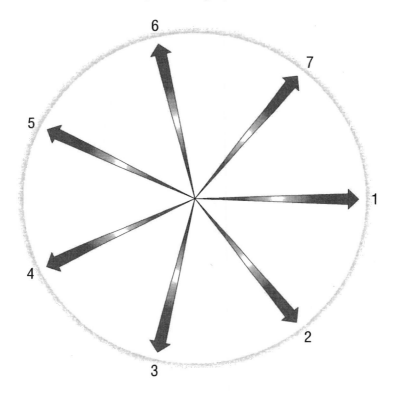

1 Balga Blackboy
2 Blue-Topped Cow Weed
3 Many-Headed Dryandra
4 Red Beak Orchid
5 Silver Princess Gum
6 Error
7 Error

AUSTRALIAN LIVING FLOWER ESSENCES

HOMEOPATHY AND ESSENCES—TABLE 2F
7. Topic: Spiritual Development

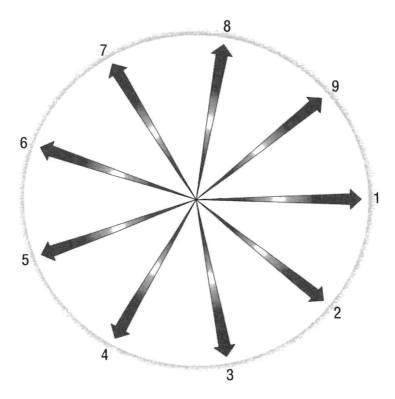

1 Goddess Grasstree
2 Green Rose
3 Purple Nymph Water Lily
4 Queensland Bottlebrush
5 West-Australian Smoke Brush
6 White Nymph Water Lily
7 Wolly Smokebrush
8 Yellow and Green Kangaroo Paw
9 Error

AUSTRALIAN LIVING FLOWER ESSENCES

HOMEOPATHY AND ESSENCES—TABLE 2F

8. Topic: Vitality, Clarity, Ability to Act

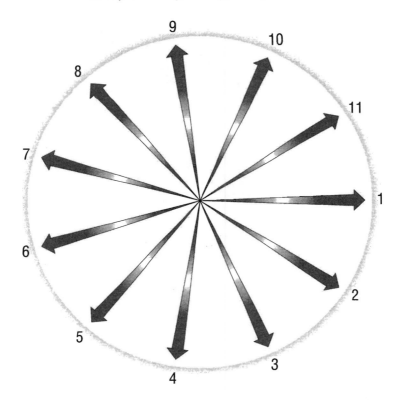

1 Leafless Orchid
2 Pink Fountain Trigger Plant
3 Pink Trumpet Flower
4 Purple Enamel Orchid
5 Snake Vine
6 White Eremophila
7 Wolly Banksia
8 Yellow Boronia
9 Yellow Flag Flower
10 Error
11 Error

137

AUSTRALIAN LIVING FLOWER ESSENCES

HOMEOPATHY AND ESSENCES—TABLE 2F

9. Topic: Social Contacts

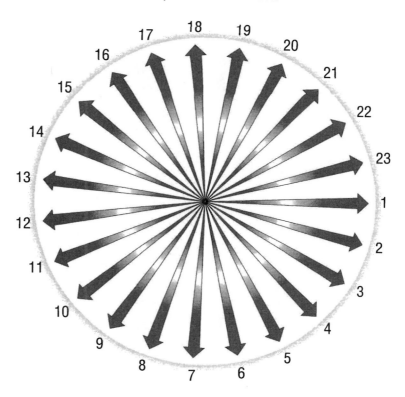

1 Blue Leschenaultia	9 Pin Cushion Hakea	15 Rose Cone Flower
2 Brachycome	10 Pixie Mops	16 Russian No. 5
3 Cat's Paw	11 Prange Spiked Pea Flower	17 Snake Bush
4 Common White Spider Orchid	12 Rabbit Orchid	18 Southern Cross
5 Cowslip Orchid	13 Red Feather Flower	19 Ursinia
6 Geraldton Wax	14 Red Leschen-aultia	20 Veronica
7 Golden Glora Grevillea		21 West-Australian Christmas Tree
8 Parakeelya		22 Error
		23 Error

AUSTRALIAN BUSH FLOWER ESSENCES

HOMEOPATHY AND ESSENCES—TABLE 2G
Group Selection Table

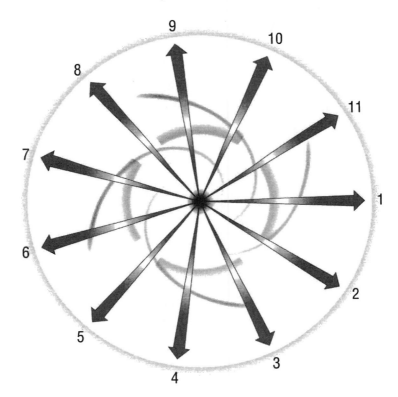

1 Authority Problems, pg. 140
2 Healing, pg. 141
3 Inner Serenity, pg. 142
4 Joy in Life/Opening Up to Life, pg. 143
5 Self-Confidance, pg. 144
6 Sexuality and Partnership, pg. 145
7 Spiritual Development, pg. 146
8 Overcoming Emotional Blocks, pg. 147
9 Vitality, Clarity, Ability to Act, pg. 148
10 Living Together with Others, pg. 149
11 Error

AUSTRALIAN BUSH FLOWER ESSENCES

HOMEOPATHY AND ESSENCES—TABLE 2G

1. Topic: Authority Problems

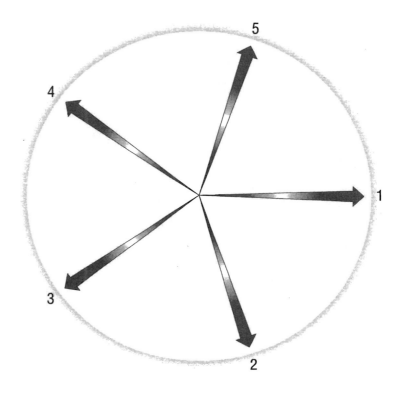

1 Red Helmet
2 Sturt Desert Pea
3 Waratah
4 Error
5 Error

AUSTRALIAN BUSH FLOWER ESSENCES

HOMEOPATHY AND ESSENCES—TABLE 2G
2. Topic: Healing

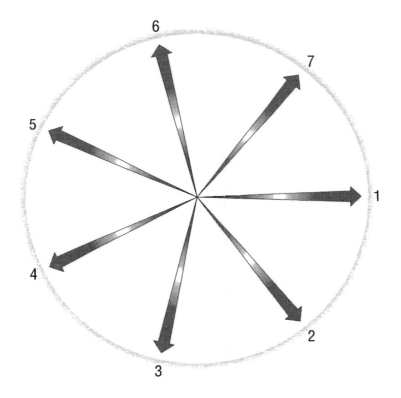

1 Bush Fuchsia
2 Fringed Violet
3 Grey Spider Flower
4 Mulla Mulla
5 She Oak
6 Spinifex
7 Error

AUSTRALIAN BUSH FLOWER ESSENCES

HOMEOPATHY AND ESSENCES—TABLE 2G

3. Topic: Inner Serenity

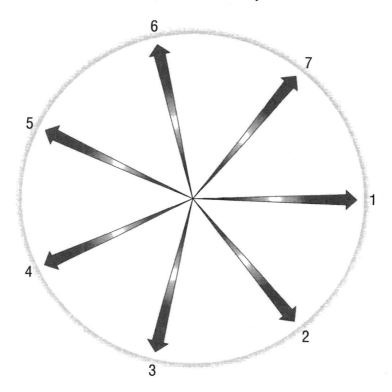

1   Black-Eyed Susan
2   Boronia
3   Crowea
4   Hibbertia
5   Tal Yellow Top
6   Error
7   Error

AUSTRALIAN BUSH FLOWER ESSENCES

HOMEOPATHY AND ESSENCES—TABLE 2G

4. Topic: Joy in Life and Opening Up to Life

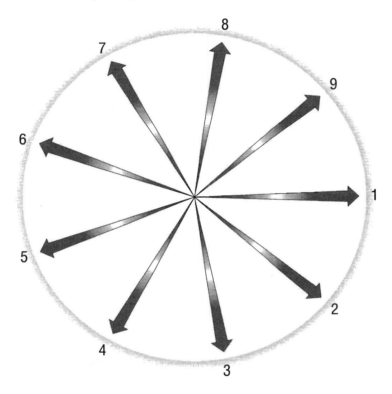

1   Bottlebrush
2   Little Flannel Flower
3   Mountain Devil
4   Red Lily
5   Silver Princess
6   Southern Cross
7   Sundew
8   Sunshine Wattle
9   Error

AUSTRALIAN BUSH FLOWER ESSENCES

HOMEOPATHY AND ESSENCES—TABLE 2G

5. Self-Confidence

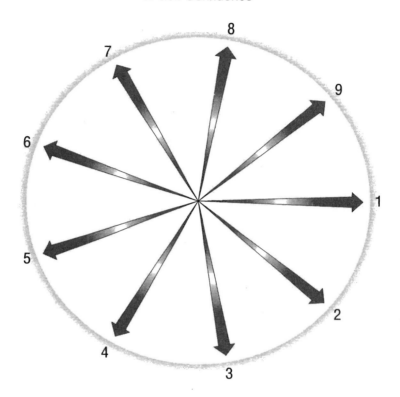

1 Dog Rose
2 Five Corners
3 Illawara Flame Tree
4 Philotheca
5 Red Grevillea
6 Sturt Desert Rose
7 Turkey Bush
8 Error
9 Error

AUSTRALIAN BUSH FLOWER ESSENCES

HOMEOPATHY AND ESSENCES—TABLE 2G

6. Topic: Sexuality and Partnership

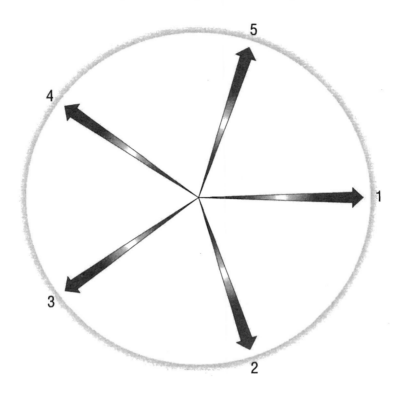

1 Billy Goat Plum
2 Bush Gardenia
3 Wisteria
4 Error
5 Error

AUSTRALIAN BUSH FLOWER ESSENCES

HOMEOPATHY AND ESSENCES—TABLE 2G

7. Topic: Spiritual Development

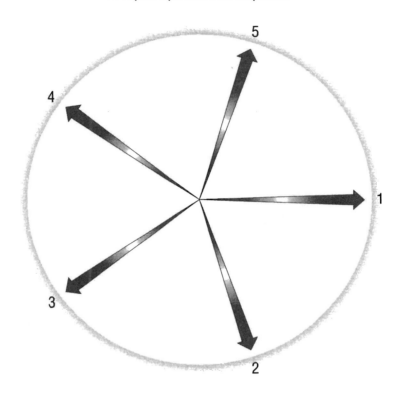

1 Bauhinia
2 Bush Iris
3 Isopogon
4 Paw Paw
5 Error

AUSTRALIAN BUSH FLOWER ESSENCES

HOMEOPATHY AND ESSENCES—TABLE 2G

8. Topic: Overcoming Emotional Blocks

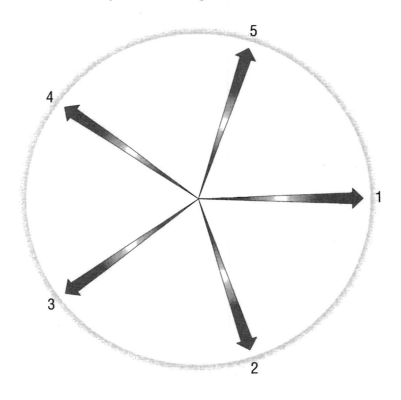

1   Bluebell
2   Dagger Hakea
3   Flannel Flower
4   Error
5   Error

AUSTRALIAN BUSH FLOWER ESSENCES

HOMEOPATHY AND ESSENCES—TABLE 2G

9. Topic: Vitality, Clarity, Ability to Act

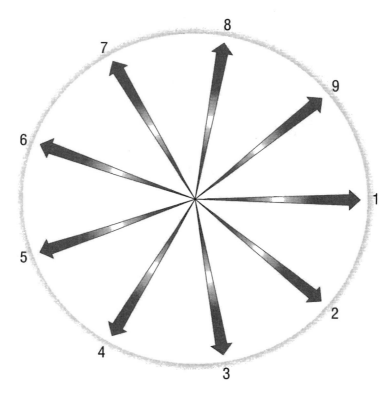

1   Banksia Robur
2   Jacaranda
3   Kapok Bush
4   Macrocarpa
5   Old Man Banksia
6   Peach Flowered Tree
7   Wild Potato Bush
8   Error
9   Error

AUSTRALIAN BUSH FLOWER ESSENCES

HOMEOPATHY AND ESSENCES—TABLE 2G

10. Topic: Living Together with Others

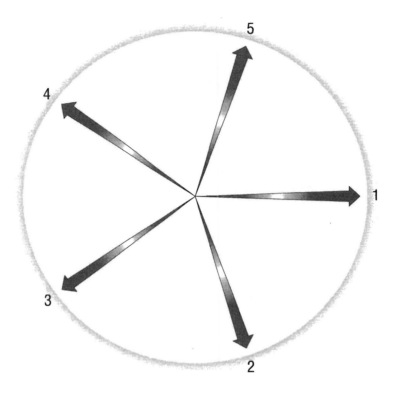

1 Kangaroo Paw
2 Slender Rice Flower
3 Wedding Bush
4 Yellow Cowslip Orchid
5 Error

ARIZONAN DESERT ESSENCES

HOMEOPATHY AND ESSENCES—TABLE 2H
Group Selection Table

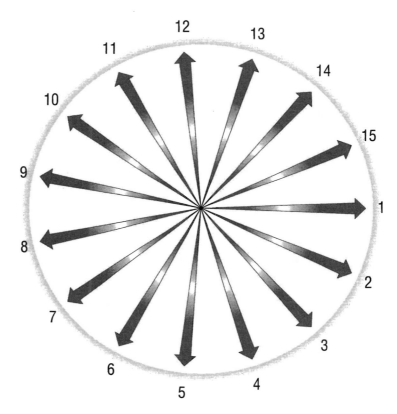

1 Sexual Identity, pg. 151
2 Setting Limits, pg. 152
3 Healing, pg. 153
4 Inner Serenity, pg. 154
5 Clarity and Ability to Act, pg. 155
6 Opening Up to Love, pg. 156
7 Self-Confidence, pg. 157
8 Sexuality and Partnership, pg. 158

9 Facing Up to Life and Trusting It, pg. 159
10 Spiritual Development, pg. 160
11 Overcoming Energy Blocks, pg. 161
12 Wisdom of Age, pg. 162
13 Living Together with Others, pg. 163
14 Error
15 Error

ARIZONAN DESERT ESSENCES

HOMEOPATHY AND ESSENCES—TABLE 2H
1. Topic: Sexual Identity

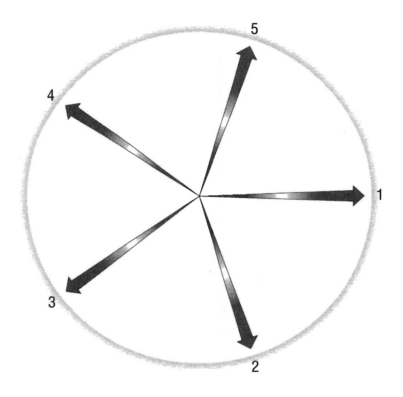

1   Mala Mujer
2   Pomegranate
3   Queen of the Night
4   Error
5   Error

ARIZONAN DESERT ESSENCES

HOMEOPATHY AND ESSENCES—TABLE 2H
2. Topic: Setting Limits

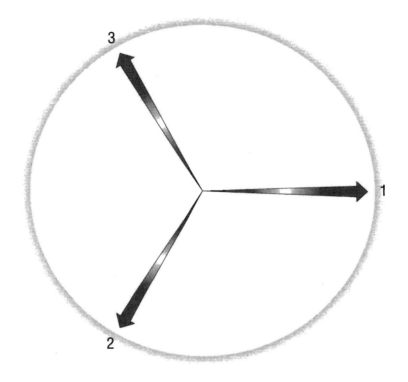

1 Bright Star
2 Desert Christmas Cholla
3 Error

ARIZONAN DESERT ESSENCES

HOMEOPATHY AND ESSENCES—TABLE 2H
3. Topic: Healing

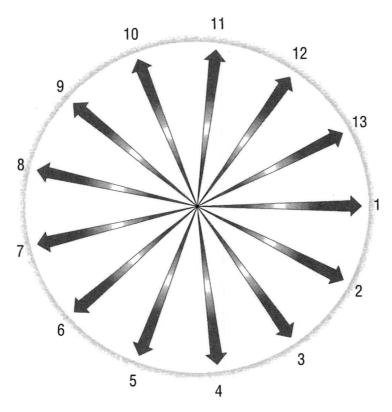

1	Aloe	8	Staghorn Cholla
2	Ephedra	9	Star Primrose
3	Fairy Duster	10	Wolfberry
4	Hackberry	11	Woven Spine
5	Immortal		Pineapple Cactus
6	Organ Pipe	12	Error
7	Scorpion Weed	13	Error

ARIZONAN DESERT ESSENCES

HOMEOPATHY AND ESSENCES—TABLE 2H
4. Topic: Inner Serenity

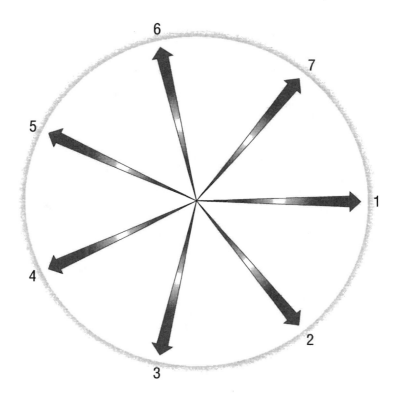

1 Bougainvillea
2 Buffalo Gourd
3 Candy Barrel Cactus
4 Foothills Paloverde
5 Melon Loco
6 Strawberry Cactus
7 Error

Arizonan Desert Essences

Homeopathy and Essences—Table 2H
5. Topic: Clarity and Ability to Act

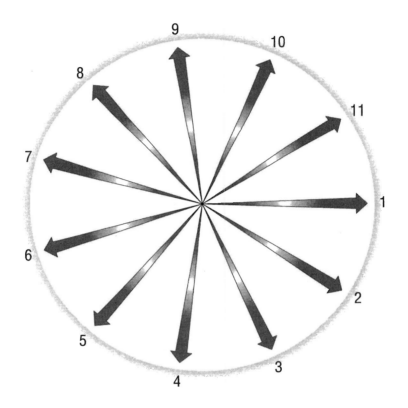

1   Cliff Rose
2   Hoptree
3   Fire Prickly Pear
4   Mariola
5   Pencil Cholla Cactus
6   Ratany
7   Soaptree Yucca
8   Spanish Bayonet Yucca
9   Syrian Rue
10 Error
11 Error

ARIZONAN DESERT ESSENCES

HOMEOPATHY AND ESSENCES—TABLE 2H
6. Topic: Opening Up to Love

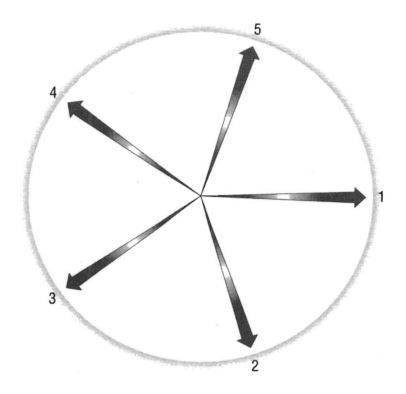

1 Desert Holly
2 Maripose Lily
3 Mesquite
4 Error
5 Error

ARIZONAN DESERT ESSENCES

HOMEOPATHY AND ESSENCES—TABLE 2H
7. Self-Confidence

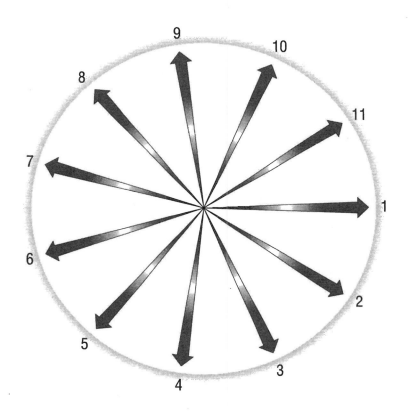

1 Agave
2 Beargrass
3 Desert Marigold
4 Evening Star
5 Mexican Star
6 Milky Nipple Cactus
7 Mullein
8 Oregon Grape
9 Spineless Prickly Pear
10 Star Leaf
11 Error

ARIZONAN DESERT ESSENCES

HOMEOPATHY AND ESSENCES—TABLE 2H
8. Topic: Sexuality and Partnership

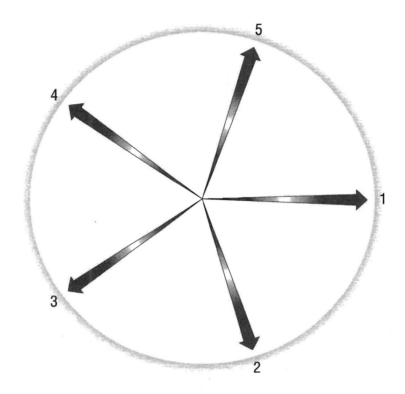

1   Big Root Jatropha
2   Bisbee Behive Cactus
3   Klein's Pencil Cholla Cactus
4   Teddy Bear Cholla Cactus
5   Error

Arizonan Desert Essences

Homeopathy and Essences—Table 2H

9. Topic: Facing Up to Life

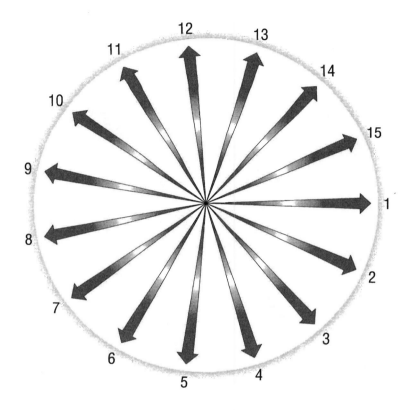

1	Arizona White Oak	9	Jumping Cholla Cactus
2	Bouvardia	10	Mexican Shell Flower
3	Camphorweed	11	Prickley Pear Cactus
4	Coral Bean	12	Saguaro
5	Crown of Thorns	13	Whitethorn
6	Damiana	14	Error
7	Desert Willow	15	Error
8	Jojoba		

ARIZONAN DESERT ESSENCES

HOMEOPATHY AND ESSENCES—TABLE 2H
10. Topic: Spiritual Development

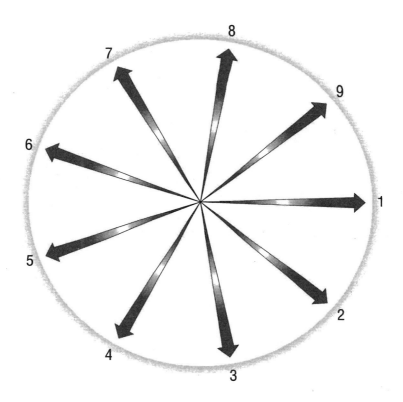

1 Cow Parsnip
2 Indian Tobacco
3 Indigo Bush
4 Mountain Mahogany
5 Sacred Datura
6 Tarbush
7 Thurber's Gilia
8 White Desert Primrose
9 Error

ARIZONAN DESERT ESSENCES

HOMEOPATHY AND ESSENCES—TABLE 2H
11. Topic: Overcoming Energy Blocks

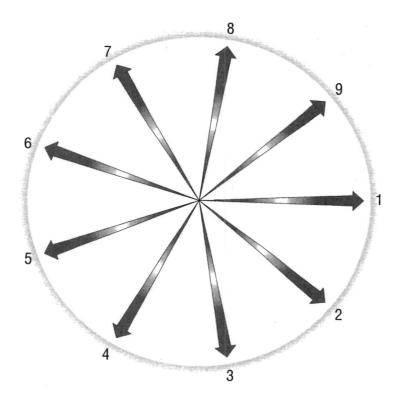

1. Cane Cholla Cactus
2. Cardon
3. Chaparral
4. Compass Barrell Cactus
5. Indian Root
6. Ocotillo
7. Rainbow Cactus
8. Violet Curis
9. Error

ARIZONAN DESERT ESSENCES

HOMEOPATHY AND ESSENCES—TABLE 2H
12. Topic: Wisdom of Age

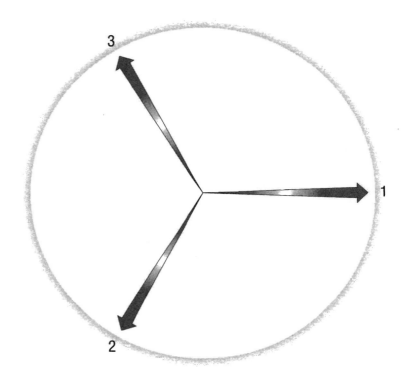

1   Senita
2   Error
3   Error

ARIZONAN DESERT ESSENCES

HOMEOPATHY AND ESSENCES—TABLE 2H

13. Topic: Living Together with Others

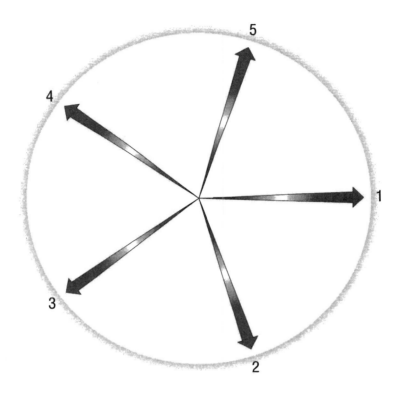

1   Devil's Claw
2   Fishhook Cactus
3   Hedgehog Cactus
4   Wild Grapevine
5   Error

PERELANDRA ESSENCES

HOMEOPATHY AND ESSENCES—TABLE 21
Group Selection Table

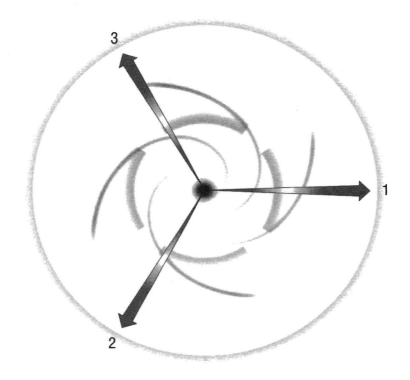

1. Garden Essences, pg. 165
2. Rose Essences, pg. 166
3. Error

PERELANDRA ESSENCES

HOMEOPATHY AND ESSENCES—TABLE 21
Perelandra Garden Essences

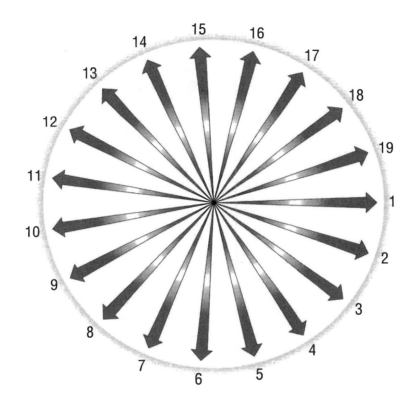

1	Broccoli	11	Salvia
2	Cauliflower	12	Snap Pea
3	Celery	13	Summer Squash
4	Chives	14	Sweet Bell Pepper
5	Comfrey	15	Tomato
6	Corn	16	Yellow Yarrow
7	Cucumber	17	Zinnia
8	Dill	18	Zucchini
9	Nasturtium	19	Error
10	Okra		

PERELANDRA ESSENCES

HOMEOPATHY AND ESSENCES—TABLE 2I
Perelandra Rose Essences

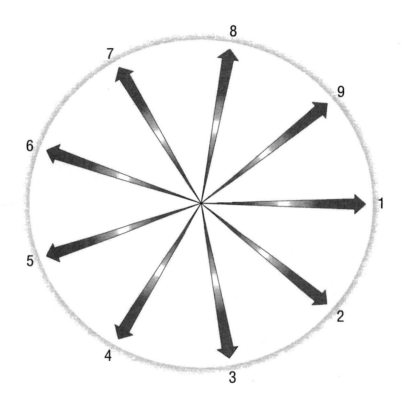

1 Ambassador
2 Eclipse
3 Gruss aus Aachen ("Greetings from Aachen")
4 Nymphenburg
5 Orange Ruffles
6 Peace
7 Royal Highness
8 White Lightning
9 Error

CALIFORNIA FLOWER ESSENCES

HOMEOPATHY AND ESSENCES—TABLE 2H
Group Selection Table

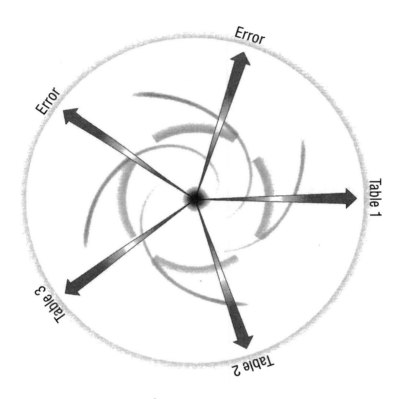

Table 1, pg. 168
Table 2, pg. 169
Table 3, pg. 170
Error
Error

CALIFORNIA FLOWER ESSENCES

HOMEOPATHY AND ESSENCES—TABLE 2H
Table 1

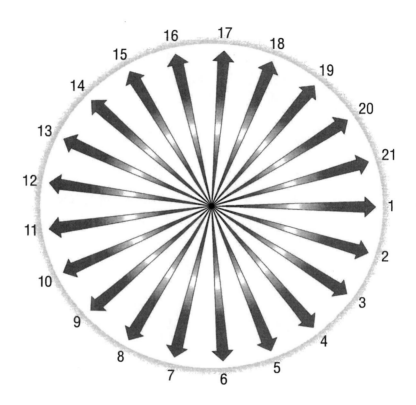

1	Aloe Vera	12	California Wild Rose
2	Arnica	13	Cayenne
3	Basil	14	Chamomile
4	Blackberry	15	Chaparral
5	Black-Eyed Susan	16	Corn
6	Bleeding Heart	17	Dandelion
7	Borage	18	Deer Brush
8	Buttercup	19	Dill
9	Calendula	20	Dogwood
10	California Pitcher Plant	21	Error
11	California Poppy		

CALIFORNIA FLOWER ESSENCES

Table 2

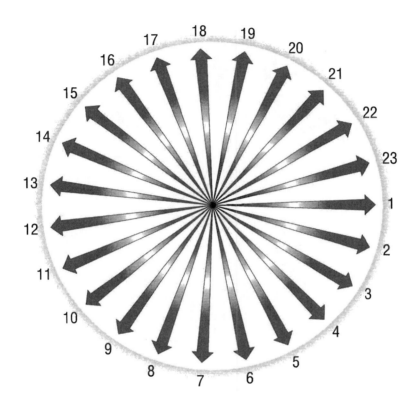

1	Filaree	13	Madia
2	Fuchsia	14	Mallow
3	Garlic	15	Manzanita
4	Golden Ear Drops	16	Mariposa Lilly
5	Goldenrod	17	Morning Glory
6	Hounds Tongue	18	Mountain Pennyroyal
7	Indian Paintbrush	19	Mountain Pride
8	Indian Pink	20	Mugwort
9	Iris	21	Mullein
10	Larkspur	22	Error
11	Lavender	23	Error
12	Lotus		

CALIFORNIA FLOWER ESSENCES

HOMEOPATHY AND ESSENCES—TABLE 2H
Table 3

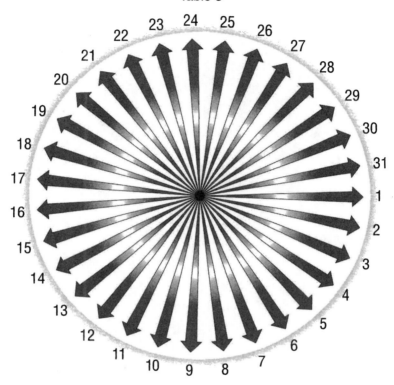

1	Nasturtium	14	Scarlet Monkey-flower
2	Oregon Grape	15	Scotch Broom
3	Penstemon	16	Self-Heal
4	Peppermint	17	Shasta-Daisy
5	Pink Yarrow	18	Shooting Star
6	Pomegranate	19	Star Thistle
7	Quaking Grass	20	Star Tulip
8	Quince	21	Sticky Monkeyflower
9	Rabbitbrush	22	Sunflower
10	Red Clover	23	Sweet Pea
11	Sagebrush	24	Tansy
12	Saguaro	25	Tiger Lily
13	Saint John's Wort		

26	Trumpet Vine
27	Violet
28	Yarrow
29	Yerba Santa
30	Zinnea
31	Error

LightBeings Master Essences

Homeopathy and Essences—Table 2K

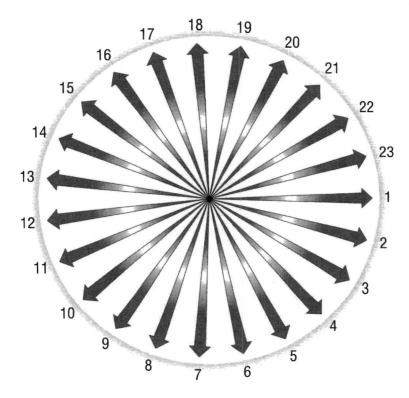

1   Maha Chohan—Inner Wisdom
2   Lao Tse—Acceptance and Inner Peace
3   El Morya—Trust
4   Kwan Yin—Dedication
5   Christ—Truth and Unconditional Love
6   Djwal Khul—Accepting Your Own Strength
7   Sanat Kumara—Connecting Heaven and Earth
8   Angelica—Transforming the Past
9   Orion—Visions
10 Kamakura—Taking Action
11 Kuthumi—Connecting with the Earth
12 Lady Nada—Being Accepted and Enjoying Life
13 Seraphis Bey—The Earthly Power
14 Victory—Growth
15 Saint Germain—Freedom
16 Hilarion—The Universal Truth
17 Pallas Athene—Joy and Abundance
18 Lady Portia—Being Balanced
19 Helion—Being Like the Sun
20 Aeolus—Recognizing the Creator within Yourself
21 Mary—Perceiving the Unity
22 Error
23 Error

SCHUESSLER SALTS

HOMEOPATHY AND ESSENCES—TABLE 3

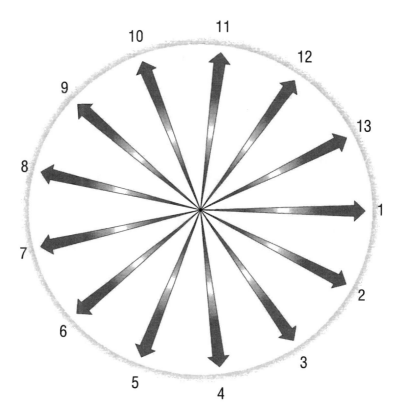

1 Ferrum phosphoricum	8 Kalium chloratum
2 Kalium phosphoricum	9 Silicea
3 Natrium phosphoricum	10 Calcium fluoratum
4 Calcium phosphoricum	11 Natrium muriaticum
5 Magnesium phosphoricum	12 Calcium sulfuricum
6 Kalium sulfuricum	13 Error
7 Natrium phosphoricum	

BIOCHEMICAL SUPPLEMENTS

HOMEOPATHY AND ESSENCES—TABLE 4

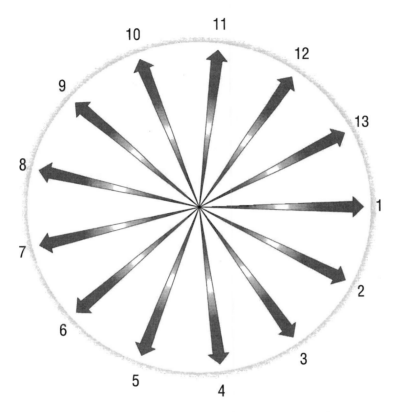

1	Arsenum jodatum	
2	Natrium bicarbonicum	
3	Calcium carbonicum	
4	Zineum chloratum	
5	Kalium aluminium-sulfuricum	
6	Cuprum arsenicosum	
7	Calcium sulfuratum	

8	Manganum sulfuricum
9	Lithium chloratum
10	Kalium jodatum
11	Kalium bromatum
12	Kalium arsenicosum
13	Error

HOMEOPATHIC MEDICINE CABINET

HOMEOPATHY AND ESSENCES
Group Selection Table

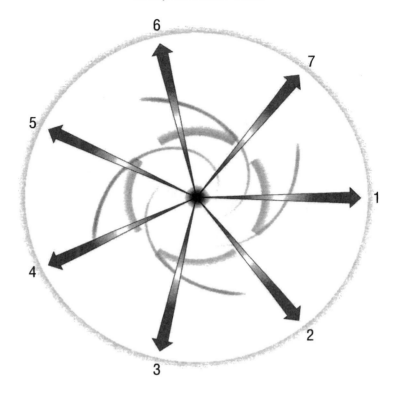

1   Table I, pg. 175
2   Table II, pg. 176
3   Table III, pg. 177
4   Table IV, pg. 178
5   Table V, pg. 179
6   Error
7   Error

HOMEOPATHIC MEDICINE CABINET

TABLE I

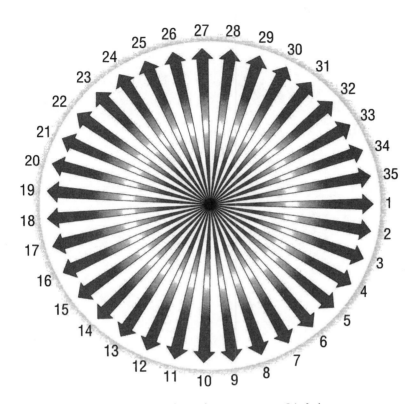

1 Abies canadensis	12 Aesculus	24 Apis
2 Abies nigra	13 Aethusa	25 Argentum metallicum
3 Abrotanum	14 Agaricus	26 Argentum nitricum
4 Absinthium	15 Agave americana	
5 Acidum aceticum	16 Agnus castus	27 Arnica
6 Acidum hydro-chloricum	17 Allium cepa	28 Arsenicum album
	18 Aloe	29 Arum triphyllum
7 Acidum lacticum	19 Alumina	30 Asa foetida
8 Acidum nitricum	20 Ambra	31 Table II
9 Acidum phospho-ricum	21 Ammonium carbonicum	32 Table III
		33 Table IV
10 Acidum sulfuri-cum	22 Anacardium	34 Table V
	23 Antimomium crudum	35 Error
11 Aconitum		

175

HOMEOPATHIC MEDICINE CABINET

TABLE II

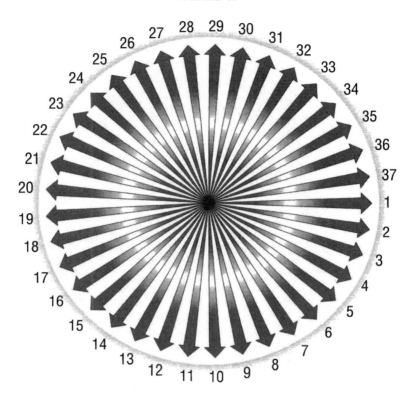

1 Aurum metallicum	12 Bufo	25 Cimicifuga
	13 Cactus	26 Cina
2 Aurum chloratum	14 Calcium carbonicum	27 Clematis
3 Avena sativa		28 Cocculus
4 Barium carbonicum	15 Calendula	29 Coccus cacti
	16 Cantharis	30 Coffea
5 Belladonna	17 Capsicum	31 Cola
6 Bellis perennis	18 Carbo animalis	32 Colchicum
7 Berberis	19 Carbo vegetabilis	33 Table I
8 Bismutum metallicum	20 Caulophyllum	34 Table III
	21 Causticum	35 Table IV
9 Borax	22 Chamomilla	36 Table V
10 Bovista	23 Chelidonium	37 Error
11 Bryonia	24 China	

HOMEOPATHIC MEDICINE CABINET

TABLE III

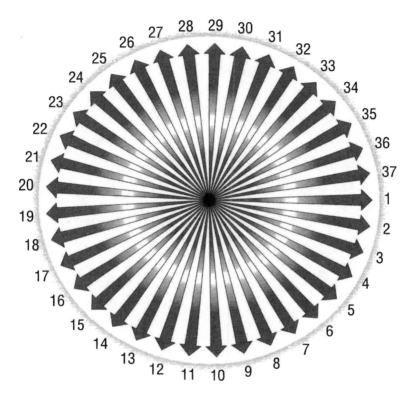

1 Colocynthis	13 Echinacea	24 Hamamelis
2 Condurango	14 Eupatorium	25 Hepar sulfuris
3 Conium	perfoliatum	26 Hydastis
4 Crataegus	15 Euphorbium	27 Hyoscyamus
5 Crotalus	16 Euphrasia	28 Hypericum
6 Cuprum arseni-	17 Ferrum metalli-	29 Ignatia
cum	cum	30 Ipecacuanha
7 Cuprum metalli-	18 Formica rufa	31 Iris versicolor
cum	19 Fucus vesiculo-	32 Jodum
8 Cyclamen	sus	33 Table I
9 Digitalis	20 Gelsemium	34 Table II
10 Dioscorea vilosa	21 Ginseng	35 Table IV
11 Drosera	22 Glonoinum	36 Table V
12 Dulcamara	23 Graphites	37 Error

HOMEOPATHIC MEDICINE CABINET

TABLE IV

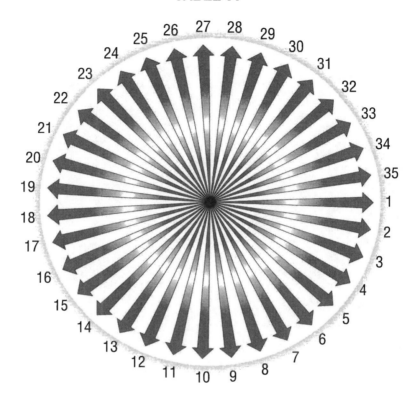

1 Kalium bichromium	12 Mandragora	25 Petroleum
2 Kalium carbonicum	13 Medorrhinum	26 Petroselinum
3 Kreosotum	14 Mercurius solubilis	27 Phosphorus
4 Lac caninum	15 Mezereum	28 Phytolacca
5 Lac defloratum	16 Millefolium	29 Plantago
6 Lachesis	17 Myristica sebifera	30 Platinum metallicum
7 Ledum	18 Naja tripudians	31 Table I
8 Lilium tigrinum	19 Naphtalinum	32 Table II
9 Luesinum	20 Nux moschata	33 Table III
10 Lycopodium	21 Nux vomica	34 Table V
11 Magnesium carbonicum	22 Oleander	35 Error
	23 Opium	
	24 Passiflora incarnata	

HOMEOPATHIC MEDICINE CABINET

TABLE V

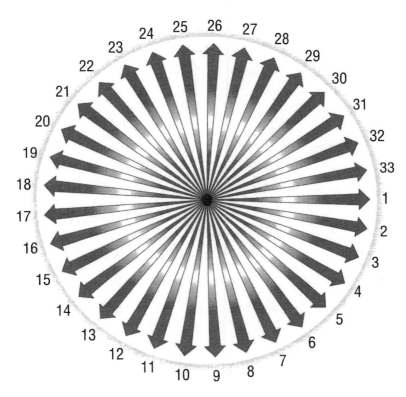

1	Plumbum metallicum	12	Spongia	24	Valeriana
2	Podophyllum	13	Stannum metallicum	25	Veratrum album
3	Psorinum	14	Staphisagria	26	Viola tricolor
4	Pulsatilla	15	Sulfur	27	Viscum album
5	Rus toxicodendron	16	Symphytum	28	Zincum metallicum
6	Sarsaparilla	17	Tabacum	29	Table I
7	Secale cornutum	18	Tarantula	30	Table II
8	Selenium	19	Taraxacum	31	Table III
9	Sepia	20	Tartarus stibiatus	32	Table IV
10	Solidago	21	Thuja	33	Error
11	Spigelia	22	Tuberculinum		
		23	Urtica		

SUPPLEMENTARY TABLE A

HOMEOPATHY AND ESSENCES

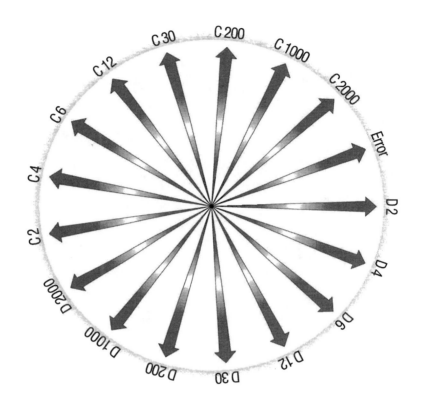

Error	C2
D2	C4
D4	C6
D6	C12
D12	C30
D30	C200
D200	C1000
D1000	C2000
D2000	

SUPPLEMENTARY TABLE B

HOMEOPATHY AND ESSENCES

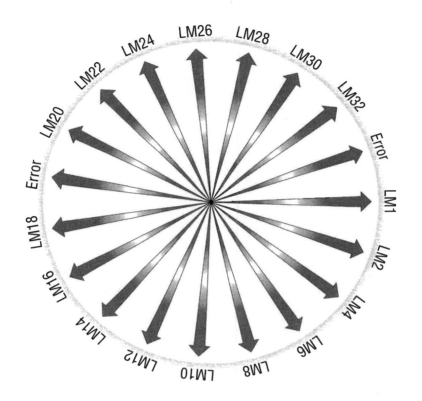

Error	LM18
LM1	Error
LM2	LM20
LM4	LM22
LM6	LM24
LM8	LM26
LM10	LM28
LM12	LM30
LM14	LM32
LM16	

SUPPLEMENTARY TABLE C

HOMEOPATHY AND ESSENCES

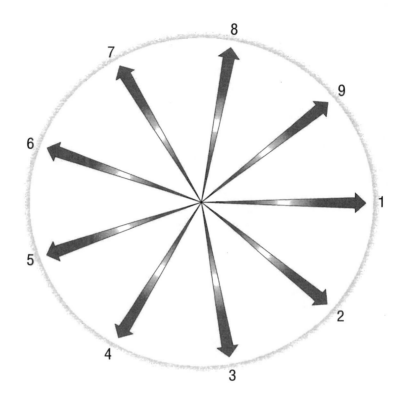

1. Rub in
2. Tablets
3. Globules
4. Error
5. Ointment
6. Rub on
7. Smell the drops
8. Drops
9. Error

SPIRITUAL GROWTH AND SELF-KNOWLEDGE

SELECTION TABLE

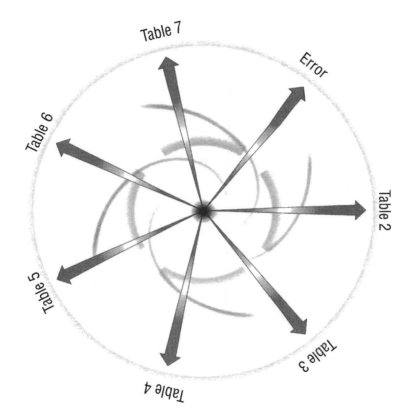

MAIN CHAKRAS

SPIRITUAL GROWTH AND SELF-KNOWLEDGE—TABLE 2

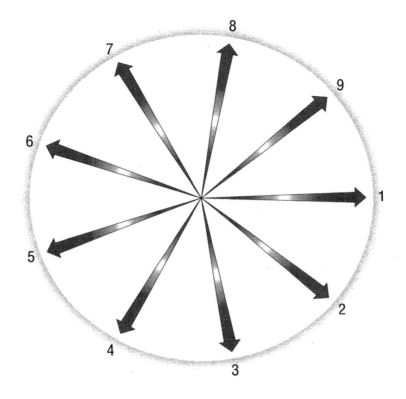

1   Root chakra
2   Sexual chakra
3   Solar plexus chakra
4   Heart chakra
5   Throat chakra
6   Forehead chakra
7   Crown chakra
8   Secondary chakras
9   Error

MERIDIANS

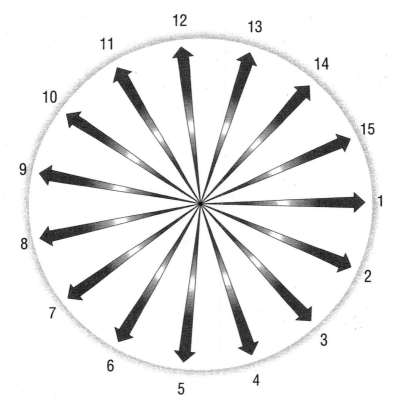

1	Liver	9	Small intestine
2	Heart	10	Stomach
3	Spleen/pancreas	11	Large intestine
4	Lungs	12	Threefold warmer
5	Kidneys	13	Conception meridian
6	Circulation/sex	14	Governor's meridian
7	Error	15	Error
8	Gallbladder		

Aura Fields

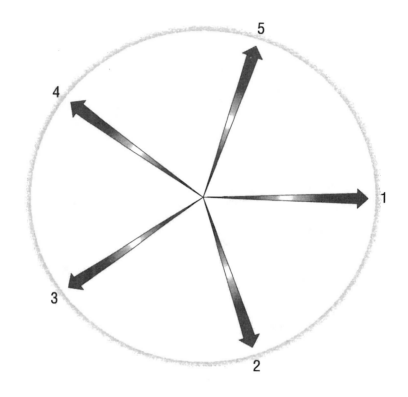

1   Ethereal body
2   Emotional body
3   Mental body
4   Spiritual body
5   Error

PATHS

SPIRITUAL GROWTH AND SELF-KNOWLEDGE—TABLE 5

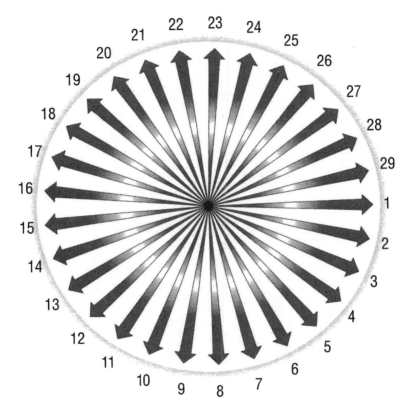

1 Reduce prejudices	11 Learn to think	23 Be as you are
2 Live love	12 Learn to feel	24 Accept your inner teacher
3 Make meaningful use of power	13 Serve	25 Accept an outer teacher
4 Pray	14 Rule	
5 Learn gratitude	15 Take on a task	26 Establish a connection to your Inner Child
6 Accept the joy of living	16 Do meaningful work	
7 Live in the here and now	17 Enter into a relationship	27 Establish a connection to your Higher Self
8 Love your body	18 Let go	28 Go into solitude
9 Love your feelings	19 Forgive	29 Error
10 See God in other people	20 Set limits	
	21 Accept	
	22 Share	

Dream Interpretation

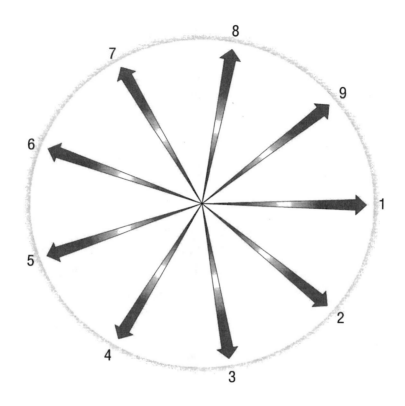

1   Future events
2   Trivial
3   Past events
4   You are your dream
5   Mental contact
6   Preparation for an experience
7   Perception
8   Processing of an experience
9   Error

ORACLES AND GUIDES

SPIRITUAL GROWTH AND SELF-KNOWLEDGE—TABLE 7

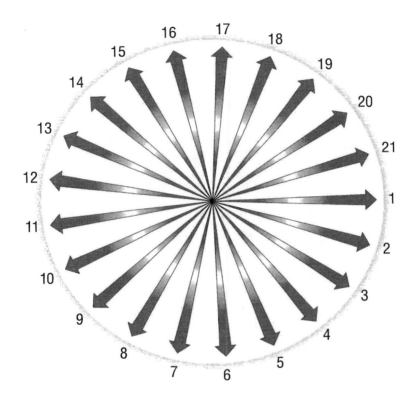

1 I Ching	12 Perceptive trance
2 Runes	13 Look into crystal ball
3 OH Cards	14 Look into mirror
4 Cards of Power	15 Read lines of hand
5 Tarot	16 Clear dreaming
6 Numerology	17 Biorhythm
7 Lay cards (scat cards)	18 Trusting the intuition
8 Use the pendulum	19 Ask a teacher
9 Channel	20 Lenormand
10 Clairvoyant	21 Error
11 Astrology	

RELATIONSHIPS AND PARTNERSHIP

SELECTION TABLE

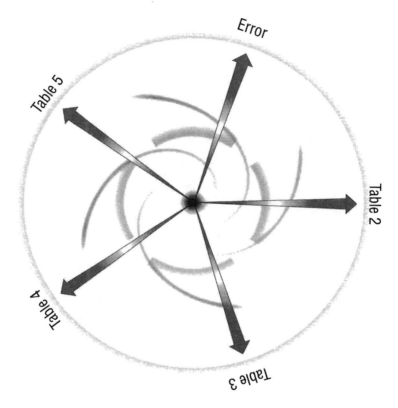

Error

Affinity/Aversion

Relationships and Partnership—Table 2

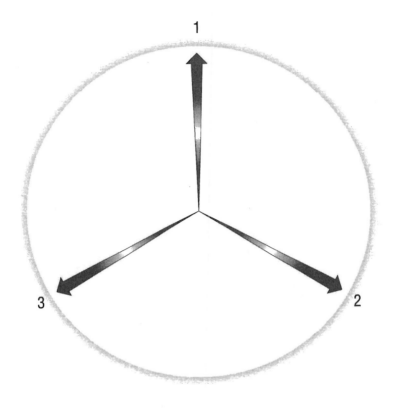

1 Aversion
2 Neutral
3 Affinity

WHAT IS THE THEME OF THE RELATIONSHIP?

RELATIONSHIPS AND PARTNERSHIP—TABLE 3

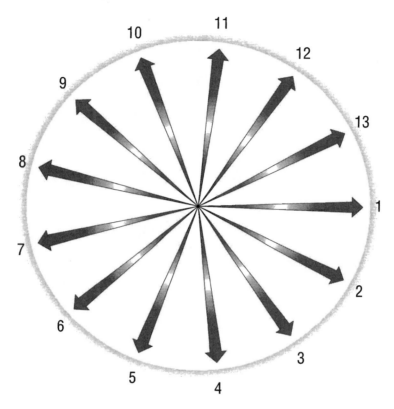

1	Work	8	Adventure
2	Love	9	Money
3	Security	10	Health
4	Facade	11	Spiritual development
5	Learning	12	Working through parental
6	Sex		transference
7	Respect	13	Error

RESOLVING PROBLEMS IN THE RELATIONSHIP

RELATIONSHIPS AND PARTNERSHIP—TABLE 4

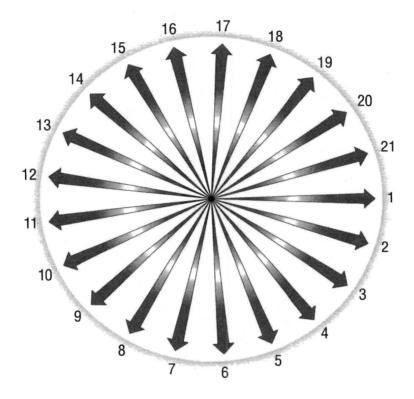

1 Couple therapy	12 Increase self-confidence
2 Individual therapy	13 Learn to fight constructively
3 Pursue mutual interests	14 Separation
4 More time for each other	15 Live together
5 Court	16 Mutual vacation
6 Set limits	17 Separate vacations
7 Let go	18 Faithfulness
8 More sex	19 Respecting the other person
9 Less sex	20 Learning to love
10 More variety in sex	21 Error
11 More eroticism	

STRAINS ON THE RELATIONSHIP/ ABILITY TO HAVE A RELATIONSHIP

RELATIONSHIPS AND PARTNERSHIP—TABLE 5

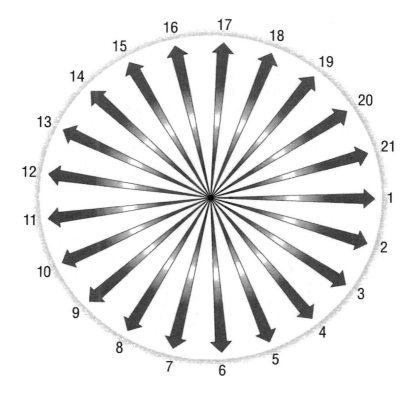

1 Superficiality	11 Sexual trauma
2 Material interest	12 Fear of closeness
3 Father projections	13 Pettiness
4 Mother projections	14 Lack of adaptability
5 Overwork	15 Living situation
6 Desire for children	16 Too many hobbies
7 Dislike of children	17 Too few mutual interests
8 Fear of commitment	18 Too little time for each other
9 Restriction of other person's freedom	19 Lack of erotic atmosphere
	20 Pride
10 Relationship to the family	21 Error

MONEY, PROFESSION, AND POSSESSIONS

SELECTION TABLE

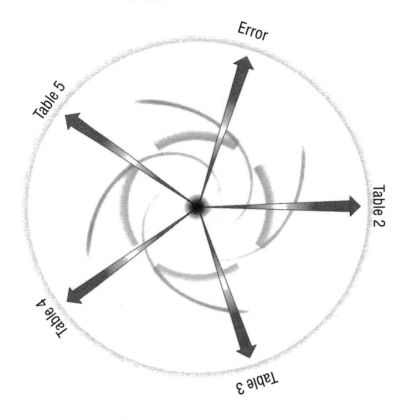

Error
Table 2—Profession, pg. 196
Table 3—Possessions, pg. 197
Table 4—Money, pg. 198
Table 5—Solving Money Problems, pg. 199

PROFESSION

MONEY, PROFESSION, AND POSSESSIONS—TABLE 2

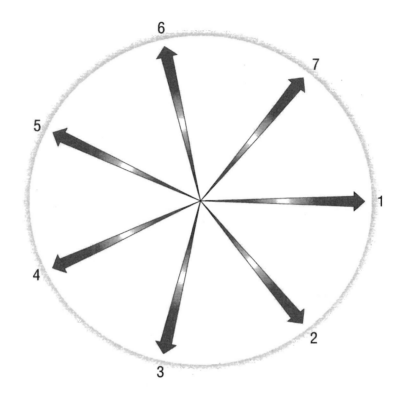

1 Change profession
2 Change job
3 Change attitude towards work
4 Advanced training
5 Accept the meaning of the work
6 Accept a sideline job
7 Error

Possessions

Money, Profession, and Possessions—Table 3

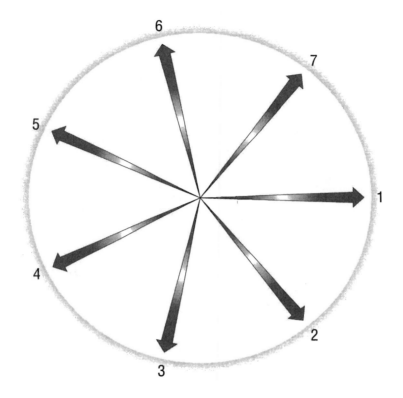

1 Understand meaning of possessions
2 Accept possessions
3 Let go of possessions
4 Share possessions
5 Defend possessions
6 Take care of possessions
7 Error

MONEY

MONEY, PROFESSION, AND POSSESSIONS—TABLE 4

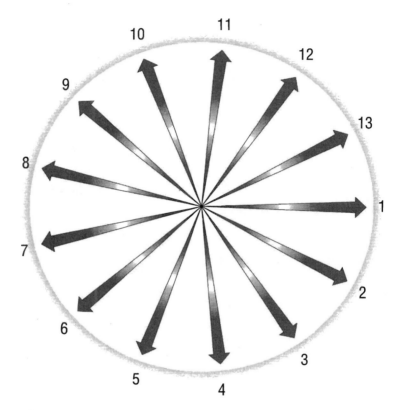

1	Understand meaning of money	8	Earn money
2	Let money flow	9	Accept new possibilities of earning money
3	Make meaningful use of money	10	Understand meaning of wealth
4	Use money for yourself	11	Understand meaning of poverty
5	Give away money	12	Spend money
6	Learn to accept money	13	Error
7	Collect money		

Solving Money Problems

Money, Profession, and Possessions—Table 5

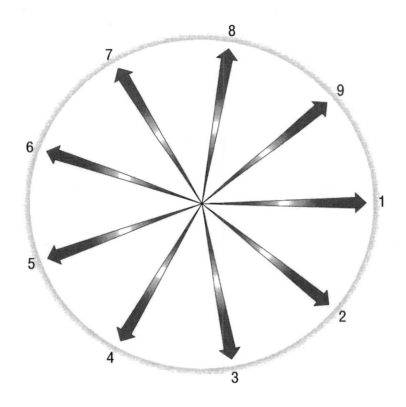

1 Learn to accept money
2 Dissolve greed
3 Accept new paths
4 Learn to live with little money
5 Learn to earn money
6 Learn to accept individual responsibility
7 Learn to transfer responsibility to others
8 Learn to budget money
9 Error

YOUR OWN PENDULUM TABLE

Topic ....

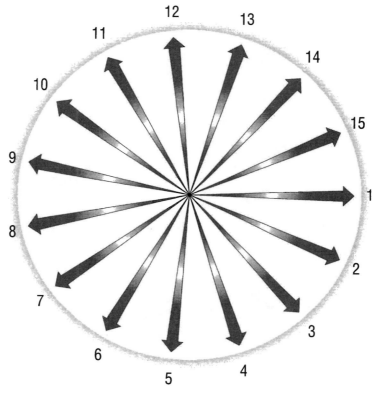

1 _____
2 _____
3 _____
4 _____
5 _____
6 _____
7 _____
8 _____

9 _____
10 _____
11 _____
12 _____
13 _____
14 _____
15 _____

YOUR OWN PENDULUM TABLE

Topic ....

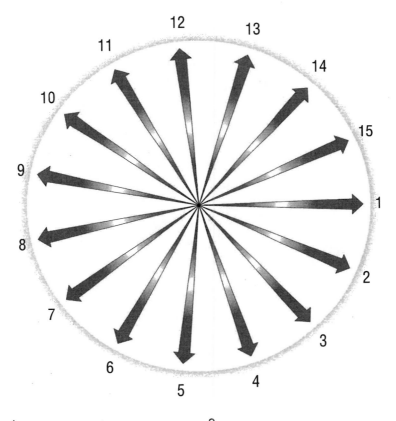

1	_____	9	_____
2	_____	10	_____
3	_____	11	_____
4	_____	12	_____
5	_____	13	_____
6	_____	14	_____
7	_____	15	_____
8	_____		

YOUR OWN PENDULUM TABLE

Topic ....

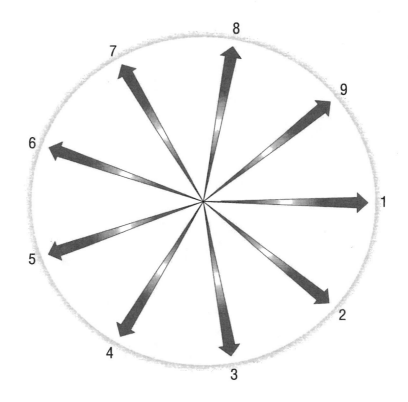

1 _____
2 _____
3 _____
4 _____
5 _____
6 _____
7 _____
8 _____
9 _____

BIBLIOGRAPHY

I. Topic: Oracles

Angel Blessings by Kimberley Marooney. Merril-West Publishing, Carmel/CA.

Runelore: A Handbook of Esoteric Runology by Edred Thorsson. Samuel Weiser Inc., York Beach/ME.

The I Ching Workbook by R. L. Wing. Doubleday & Co.

I Ching: The Book of Change by John Blofeld. George Allen & Unwin Publ. Ltd.

Medicine Cards: The Discovery of Power Through the Ways of Animals by Jamie Sams/David Carson. Bear & Co., Santa Fe/New Mexico.

The Numerology Workbook by Julia Line. The Aquarian Press, UK.

Numerology for the New Age by Lynn Buess. DeVorss & Co., CA.

II. Topic: Using the Pendulum, Radiesthesia, and Feng Shui

Dowsing: Techniques and Applications by Tom Graves. Turnstone Books, London.

Beyond Pendulum Power: Entering the Energy World by Greg Nielsen. Conscious Books, Reno/Nevada.

Living Color by Sarah Rossbach/Lin Yun. Kodansah International, New York. (Feng Shui)

The Feng Shui Handbook by Derek Walters. The Aquarian Press, UK.

III. Topic: Colors

The Colours of Your Mind by Gerry Rhodes/Sue Thame. William Collins, Sons & Co., London.

IV. Topic: Chakras and Subtle Energy Systems

The Chakra Handbook by Baginsky/Sharamon. Lotus Light/ Shangrila.

The Chakras and the Human Energy Fields by Dora van Gelder-Kunz/Shafica Karagulla. Theosophical Publ. House.

The Body of Light by John Mann/Lar Short. Globe Press Books.

V. Topic: Nutrition

Nourishing Wisdom: A New Understanding of Eating by Marc David. Harmony Books, NY.

Magic in Food by Scott Cunningham. Llewellyn Publ., St. Paul/MN.

VI. Topic: Meditation

Hearts on Fire: The Tao of Meditation by Stephen Wolinsky. Blue Dove Press.

The Way of ZEN by Alan Watts. Pantheon Books Inc.

The Orange Book by Osho. Neo-Sannyas Intern.

VII. Topic: Alternative Therapies

Homeopathy: Heart & Soul: Treatment for Emotional Problems by Keith Souter. The C.W. Daniel Co. Ltd, UK.

The Complete System of Self-Healing by Stephen T. Chang. Tao Publ., San Francisco/CA.

The Complete Crystal Guidebook by Uma Silbey. U-Read Publ., San Francisco/CA.

Flower Essences of Alaska by Steve Johnson. The Alaskan Flower Project, Homer/Alaska.

Subtle Aromatherapy by Patricia David. C.W. Daniel Co. Ltd.

Ayurveda: Secrets of Healing by Maya Tiwari. Lotus Press, Twin Lakes/WI.

Aromatherapy by Daniele Ryman. Piatkus Publ., London.
The Complete Reiki Handbook by Walter Lübeck. Lotus Light/Shangrila.
Reiki For First Aid by Walter Lübeck. Lotus Light/Shangrila.
Reiki—Way of the Heart by Walter Lübeck. Lotus Light/Shangrila.
Rainbow Reiki by Walter Lübeck. Lotus Light/Shangrila.
Shamanic Experience by Kenneth Meadows. Element Inc.
Essiac: A Native Herbal Cancer Remedy by Cynthia B. Olsen. Kali Press, Pagosa Springs/Colorado.
Healing the Mind by Bill Moyers (Ed.). Doubleday.
The Healing Power of Grapefruit Seed by Baginski/Sharamon. Lotus Light/Shangrila.
Zen-Shiatsu by Shitsuto Masunaga/Wataru Ohaski. Japan Publications Inc.

VIII.Topic: Spiritual Growth

Spiritwalker by Hank Wesselmann. Bantam Books.
The Celestine Prophecy: An Adventure by James Redfield.
The Essence of Allan Watts by Allan Watts. Celestial Arts, CA.
Ectasy Is a New Frequency by Chris Griscom. Bear & Co., Santa Fe/New Mexico.

IX.Topic: Relationships

Sex in Human Loving by Eric Berne. Simon and Schuster, NY.
Myth and Sexuality by Jamake Highwater. NAL Books.
The Evolution of Desire—Strategies of Human Mating by David M. Buss. Basic Books, New York.

ABOUT THE AUTHOR

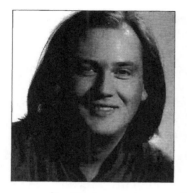

Walter Lübeck is a renowned Reiki master, founder and director of the Reiki-Do Institute. He is a bestselling prolific author of classic works on Reiki, as well as books on other healing methods, such as work with Chakra balancing, pendulums, and auras. In the last years he has developed a method he refers to as Rainbow Reiki which includes an unlimited spectrum of applications like channeling, astral travel, making Reiki essences, therapy with precious stones, as well as personality development and wholistic enviromental protection. He has spent many years studying diverse martial arts, meditation, natural healing and energy work of all kinds. Walter Lübeck orients himself in his entire work toward three basic principles: support of personal individual responsibility, development of the ability to love, and conciousness expansion. His goal is to contribute to the betterment of the quality of daily life through spiritual knowledge and thereby to bring man, nature and God in harmony. He lives in Weserbergland, Germany, in a landscape filled with ancient power spots.

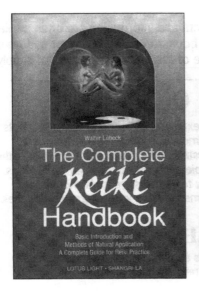

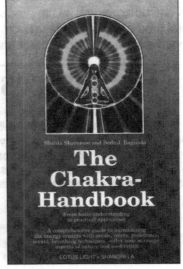

Walter Lübeck

The Complete Reiki Handbook

Basic Introduction and Methods of Natural Application—A Complete Guide for Reiki Practice

This handbook is a complete guide for Reiki practice and a wonderful tool for the necessary adjustment to the changes inherent in a new age. The author's style of natural simplicity, much appreciated by the readers of his many bestselling books, wonderfully complements this basic method for accessing universal life energy. He shares with us, as only a Reiki master can, the personal experience accumulated in his years of practice. Lovely illustrations of the different positions make the information as easily accessible visually as the author's direct and undogmatic style of writing. This work also offers a synthesis of Reiki and many other popular forms of healing.

192 pages, $ 14.95

Shalila Sharamon and Bodo J. Baginski

The Chakra Handbook

From Basic Understanding to Practical Application

Knowledge of the energy centers provides us with deep, comprehensive insight into the effects the subtle powers have on the human organism. This book vividly describes the functioning of the energy centers. For practical work with the chakras this book offers a wealth of possibilities: the use of sounds, colors, gemstones, and fragrances with their own specific effects, augmented by meditation, breathing techniques, foot reflexology massage of the chakra points, and the instilling of universal life energy. The description of nature experiences, yoga practices, and the relationship of each indiviual chakra to the zodiac additionally provides inspiring and valuable insight.

192 pages, $ 14.95

Herbs and other natural health products and information are often available at natural food stores or metaphysical bookstores. If you cannot find what you need locally, you can contact one of the following sources of supply.

Sources of Supply:

The following companies have an extensive selection of useful products and a long track-record of fulfillment. They have natural body care, aromatherapy, flower essences, crystals and tumbled stones, homeopathy, herbal products, vitamins and supplements, videos, books, audio tapes, candles, incense and bulk herbs, teas, massage tools and products and numerous alternative health items across a wide range of categories.

WHOLESALE:

Wholesale suppliers sell to stores and practitioners, not to individual consumers buying for their own personal use. Individual consumers should contact the RETAIL supplier listed below. Wholesale accounts should contact with business name, resale number or practitioner license in order to obtain a wholesale catalog and set up an account.

Lotus Light Enterprises, Inc.

PO Box 1008 PE
Silver Lake, WI 53170 USA
262 889 8501 (phone)
262 889 8591 (fax)
800 548 3824 (toll free order line)

RETAIL:

Retail suppliers provide products by mail order direct to consumers for their personal use. Stores or practitioners should contact the wholesale supplier listed above.

Internatural

PO Box 489 PE
Twin Lakes, WI 53181 USA
800 643 4221 (toll free order line)
262 889 8581 office phone
EMAIL: internatural@internatural.com
WEB SITE: www.internatural.com

Web site includes an extensive annotated catalog of more than 14,000 items that can be ordered "on line" for your convenience 24 hours a day, 7 days a week.